To my colleague and
best friend Tony
Visit to Canada May 2006.

Ron

Real Friends Tony & Sybil
for an unforgetable time
in the Rockies
Love & thanks
Ron

The Royal College
of Surgeons *of* England

200 Years of History at the Millennium

John P Blandy and John S P Lumley, Editors

Published by the Royal College of Surgeons of England and Blackwell Science Ltd.

Royal College of Surgeons of England
35-43 Lincoln's Inn Fields, London WC2A 3PN
Tel: 020 7405 3474 Fax: 020 7831 9438
http://www.rcseng.ac.uk

Blackwell Science Ltd
Osney Mead, Oxford OX2 0EL
http://www.blackwell-science.com

Distributors in the UK:
Marston Book Services Ltd
PO Box 269
Abingdon, Oxon OX14 4YN
Tel: (orders) 01235 465500 Fax: 01235 465555

First published 2000.
ISBN 0 632 05396 8

Designed and typeset by Chatland Sayer, London.
Printed and bound in Italy by Rotolito Lombarda SpA, Milan.

A catalogue record for this title is available from the British Library.

Blackwell
Science

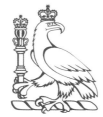

Contents

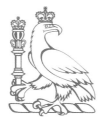

Foreword

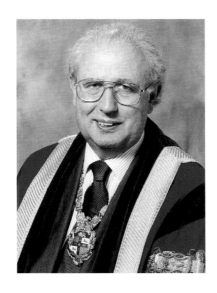

A birthday is always a time for celebration; a 200th birthday is a time for very special celebration and commemoration.

When Council gave initial thought as to how the College Bicentenary should be celebrated, the concept of a richly illustrated history of the College was one of the first suggestions to gain favour – this book is the result. It differs markedly both from the commemorative history issued at our Centenary in 1900, and from the College history written by Zachary Cope and conceived at the time of our 150th anniversary. Apart from the benefits of modern graphic design and colour printing, the present volume encompasses in reader-friendly fashion the truly enormous changes that have taken place within and without the College over the past few decades, as well as our earlier history. It includes chapters on the Faculties, our close relationship with the specialist associations, and our many treasures, as well as giving an overview of the important role the College plays within British surgery as we enter the 21st century.

The editors are to be congratulated on pruning and blending the enormous amount of submitted material, both written and visual, into an attractive, readable volume that I know will give great pleasure to many.

Barry Jackson

President, January 2000

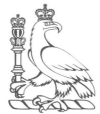

Introduction

The Royal College of Surgeons of England is not just a building in Lincoln's Inn Fields in London; it is a vigorous living entity which, like most other ancient institutions with roots in the past, has survived because it has been capable of adapting to change as new objectives and requirements have been identified year by year.

It is a uniquely English institution. It evolved from a small medieval Fellowship of Surgeons who were always closely associated with the Barbers but preserved their identity within the Company of Barber-Surgeons when providing surgeons for the armed forces of the crown. It has been an examining body for most of its history, but only more recently has it been recognised that the College should teach and educate those it examines. In the 20th century it accepted that research into surgery was one of its responsibilities, although ever since its foundation – when it accepted the custodianship of the Hunterian Collection of museum specimens built up by one of the foremost surgical research workers of all time – the College fostered research into the fields of natural history and comparative anatomy which had been among the many interests of John Hunter.

After the First World War, driven by Lord Moynihan's appreciation of the value of surgical research, the College became the centre for surgical research in the British Isles. Animal laboratories were set up in the Buckston Browne farm at Downe which, for many years, offered unique facilities for research. The College attracted teachers of the calibre of Lord Adrian, the neurophysiologist, and John Vane, the pharmacologist, both to become Nobel laureates. Good teachers became increasingly important as the College began to undertake more teaching in response to the demand for surgeons arising from two world wars. At first the College courses were in the basic sciences relevant to surgery, but soon clinical courses were needed, and the College found itself at the centre of a network of hospitals combining to provide teaching in clinical surgery.

Formal courses can only be a part of training, for a young surgeon has to learn many practical skills on the job. As a consequence the College began to inspect every junior post that purported to provide training. This required two things: a nation-wide system for the inspection of training posts and a network of College advisers and tutors to offer guidance to the trainee. In turn, this led to a system of distance learning by which young surgeons all over the country can be guided in their reading and helped in the study of the branch of surgery in which they are working. In these ways, the College has become a vital organisation which provides help, guidance and education to all its Members and Fellows.

As for research, the College today recognises that the issues that concern surgery are best investigated in hospitals where unanswerable questions regularly crop up at the operating table and the bedside. Hence, rather than pursuing surgical research in-house, the College sponsors a large number of Research Fellowships, awarded in competition, whose winners carry out their projects in university departments of surgery throughout the country and abroad. Never before has surgical research been so active or so productive.

Recently the College has assumed an active role in audit. This involves the meticulous recording of results and their comparison between centres. This, and the National Confidential Enquiry into Peri-operative Deaths (NCEPOD), which is run jointly by the College, the Royal College of Anaesthetists and the specialist associations, provides a nation-wide audit that is unique in the world. It is not always appreciated that the College has been one of the pioneers in this type of audit.

The common trunk of 'surgery in general' keeps putting out new branches, usually in response to technological advances: inert metals for mending bone, immunosuppressive drugs that make transplantation possible, endoscopes which allow major surgery to be carried out through minimal incisions. Each branch of surgery in turn sends out shoots and each shoot its set of twigs. The old orthodoxy that every surgeon should be capable of every operation has long disappeared. Rather than resist the advance of surgical specialisation, the College today is proud to house the various specialist associations within its building.

The fabric of the College has an interesting story to tell. Much of the architecture is of interest to the cognoscenti, and Members and Fellows prize three of its greatest treasures – the Nuffield College, the Library and the Hunterian Collection.

The Nuffield College began as spartan accommodation for young surgeons from the Commonwealth seeking the courses which in those days only the College could provide. Today it offers extremely comfortable residential facilities for out-of-town Members and Fellows who visit the College to teach or attend courses.

The Library comprises a unique historical collection relating to surgery which is housed in a magnificent 19th century room designed by Charles Barry, and a working library furnished with up-to-date technology allowing out-of-town Members and Fellows to check surgical literature at the computer keyboard.

At the heart of the College is sited the great Hunterian Collection which lives on, despite severe bomb damage during the Second World War, thanks to successive generations of Trustees who have protected and cherished it down the years. One of the Trustees is always the Prime Minister, a reminder that it was Parliament who purchased the Collection to be held in trust for the nation.

Despite its long history there are still misconceptions about the College. Although governments often turn to it for advice, it is independent of any government. It has had professors since its inception, but is not part of a university. It regulates the training of surgeons for the National Health Service, but is not part of that service. Unlike the British Medical Association, it is not a trade union; the College stands apart from matters relating to pay or conditions of service unless it finds them impinging on the training of surgeons, when it is obliged to speak up. Unlike the General Medical Council, the College has no statutory disciplinary powers although it is often blamed when any of its Fellows are alleged to fall below an acceptable standard of competence. In order to clarify its role within the greater medical scene, the College Council recently agreed upon a mission statement with which it is appropriate to conclude this brief introduction to 200 years of history:

The Royal College of Surgeons of England is an independent professional body committed to promoting and advancing the highest standards of surgical care for patients.

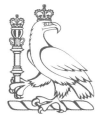

CHAPTER 1

The Fellowship *of* Surgeons

1.1 Trepanation, one of the oldest surgical operations

In this medieval scene, the surgeon appears to be removing debris from a freshly drilled hole in the cranium.

BL Sloane MSS 1977 folio 2r (Courtesy British Library)

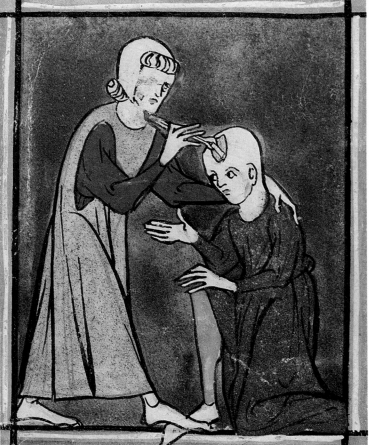

1.1

The earliest records of Greece and Rome refer to surgeons as being distinct from physicians, engaged in opening abscesses, setting fractures and dealing with wounds. One of their main occupations through to medieval times, and undoubtedly their main source of income, was the letting of blood. Different methods were used: cutting open a vein with a sharp knife or fleam, putting a heated cup over scarified skin and letting it cool, or applying leeches. Occasionally, medieval surgeons also performed the so-called 'capital operations': amputation, lithotomy and trepanation (Fig 1.1).

In times of war and in the medieval joust, surgeons' skills in dealing with fractures and wounds caused by sword, spear or arrow were highly esteemed and richly rewarded (Fig 1.2).

1.2 Removing an arrow

This scene shows the removal of a barbed arrow from a 13th century edition of the surgical treatise of Roger Frugard. The treatise recommends that the barbs of the arrowhead should be taken in a pair of forceps and pressed so that they are bent flush with the shaft, thereby facilitating withdrawal of the arrow.

Trinity College, Cambridge, MS 0.1.20
(Courtesy Trinity College, Cambridge)

1.3 John of Arderne (1306–1390)

John of Arderne was a surgeon in charge of the medical team supplied by the Fellowship of Surgeons for the expeditionary force that Edward III led to the battle of Crécy in the early 14th century. It was at Crécy that cannons introduced a terrifying new kind of pathology. Unlike the clean incision of a sword or arrow, gunshot created wounds that were crushed and easily contaminated; infection was virtually inevitable. Hence, the belief arose that gunpowder was poisonous, leading to the seemingly logical conclusion that all gunshot wounds should be cauterised. John of Arderne was also famous for his operations on fistula-in-ano, on which he wrote a treatise.

(Courtesy Wellcome Institute Library, London)

Outside large towns minor surgical procedures such as letting blood, extracting teeth or lancing abscesses were also undertaken by the village barber. The surgeon, as distinct from the barber, was denoted by the title 'leech', an honorific designation possibly deriving from their principal role as blood-letters. An example of a medieval 'leech' was John of Arderne (Fig 1.3).

The precise origins of the formal organisation of both barbers and surgeons are difficult to trace. There were fewer leeches than village barbers, but in London they were sufficient in number to form a Fellowship of Surgeons as early as 1300, as evidenced by the summons of the Fellowship by the Mayor and Aldermen to assess the accreditation of one 'Peter the Surgeon'. Though not a livery company, the Fellowship did obtain from the Mayor and Aldermen some control over the practice of surgery in the City. There also exists a record of the oath administered when swearing in three new Master Surgeons in the City of London in 1369: John Dunheved, John Hyndstoke and Nicholas Kyldesby.

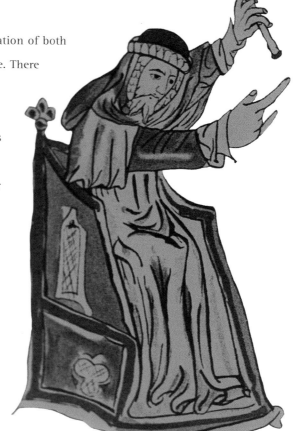

1.3

1.4 Thomas Morsted's note on an operation performed by John Bradmore

In 1403, Bradmore accompanied Henry IV at the Battle of Shrewsbury, where the King defeated the rebellion of the Percys. During the battle, one of the casualties was Prince Hal, later Henry V. The 15-year-old Prince refused to withdraw from the field of battle, saying 'Lead me thus wounded to the front line that I may, as a Prince should, kindle our fighting men with deeds not words'. Prince Hal went on to lead the charge that broke the enemy, although his wound was not by any means a 'shallow scratch': he had been hit by an arrow in the left maxilla. As often happened, the shaft came away leaving the arrowhead deep in the wound. Later that evening, Bradmore was summoned to where the Prince lay in Kenilworth Castle. He took with him his assistant, Thomas Morsted, who wrote down what he observed. In the note, preserved in the British Museum, Morsted described how Bradmore 'had out the arrowhead with an instrument made in the manner of a tongs' and proceeded to draw the tongs in the text. Afterwards the wound was 'washed with wine and cleansed with ointment'. A week later the 'place was healed with unguentum fuscum chirurgicum' – the black surgical ointment applied with a spatula.

BL. Harl. 1736 fos 41–52
(Courtesy British Library)

In 1308, the first recorded Master of the Company of Barbers was sworn in at Guildhall. For most of the 14th century, minor surgery was still in the hands of barbers whose Company complained formally in 1376 of 'country folk who come to London and without training intermeddle with barbery, surgery and the cure of maladies'. In 1388 the Company of Barbers – together with all the other guilds in the City – were required by Richard II to file returns of their organisation and property, and thus were officially listed. Two years later, the Lord Mayor admitted another four Master Surgeons into the Fellowship of Surgeons, among them John Bradmore, who was Leech to Henry IV (Fig 1.4).

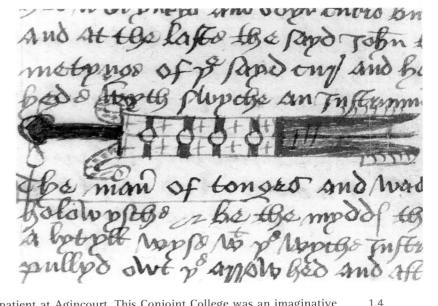

1.4

Thomas Morsted (Fig 1.5), the successor to Bradmore, established in 1423 a Conjoint College of Physicians and Surgeons, thanks largely to the influence of Humphrey, Duke of Gloucester, Morsted's patient at Agincourt. This Conjoint College was an imaginative venture; it would have put surgeons on an equal rank with physicians, and might have introduced a whole new concept of collaboration between the two ancient branches of medicine. Unfortunately, it did not survive more than a year.

1.5 Thomas Morsted's coat of arms

Thomas Morsted, Leech to Henry V, led a team of 12 surgeons to Agincourt, where he drew the pay of 30 men-at-arms and was assigned a personal bodyguard of three archers. His varlets (assistants) received the pay of an archer: sixpence a day. During the Battle of Agincourt, Humphrey, Duke of Gloucester, was stabbed. The King stood over his brother and held off the attackers; later, the Duke was dragged to safety, where he was tended by Morsted. Morsted was rewarded by the lucrative post of 'searcher' of vessels passing up and down the Thames, ie customs officer. He married the Lord Mayor's wealthy widow in 1424 and invested extensively in property, acquiring the Manor of Wotton in Surrey.

Morsted's textbook advises his assistants to have 'goodness of countenance and face, shapely of body, small fingers, steadfast hands not trembling, clear sight, be bold and hardy in sickness, gracious to sick folk, merciful to poor folk and not covetous but reasonable considering his labour and the wealth or poverty of the patient'.

BL. Harl, 1736. Mesue Englished fos. 6–14

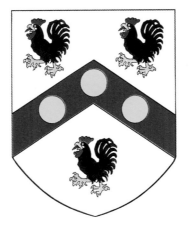

The Fellowship of Surgeons in London never numbered more than 20 members, far too few to form a guild of their own. In 1435, new ordinances drawn up by Morsted were granted to the Fellowship of Surgeons, ensuring that the small group retained its identity. The Barbers meanwhile flourished: in 1451, they were granted a coat of arms, and in 1462 a Charter of Incorporation, which was concerned primarily with surgery (probably to establish the Company of Barbers as the official body governing the practice of surgery in London).

In 1492, the Fellowship of Surgeons was called upon by Henry VII to join his expeditionary force in besieging Boulogne. They reminded the sovereign that it was customary that leeches be exempt from bearing arms. In the event, the Boulogne force never had to fight. The King of France bought off Henry VII, who returned laden with treasure. He rewarded the Fellowship of Surgeons with a 'cognizance', a heraldic badge of somewhat lower standing than the coat of arms of the Barbers (Fig 1.6).

The following year the Company of Barbers and the Fellowship of Surgeons signed an agreement under the terms of which the barbers were to refrain from the practice of surgery (except for drawing teeth) and the surgeons from shaving and hair-cutting. This agreement formalised existing arrangements, whereby the Fellowship of Surgeons retained their distinct identity.

1.6 The cognizance granted by Henry VII

Depicted on the cognizance is a rose crowned in gold. On top is the spatula for applying ointment, which was then an important surgical implement.

(Courtesy Worshipful Company of Barbers)

When Henry VIII came to the throne in 1509, this arrangement was still in force. The Barbers obtained a new charter from the King in 1512 in which he was described as their patron. It was probably then that the King gave the Barbers the beautiful silver-gilt instrument case that is preserved today (Fig 1.7). It bears on one side the coat of arms of the Barbers and on the other the cognizance of the Fellowship of Surgeons.

1.7

1.7 Surgical instrument case

The case was probably given by Henry VIII to the Company of Barbers in 1512 at the time of granting the Charter.

(Courtesy Worshipful Company of Barbers)

A milestone in the relationship of the Company of Barbers and the Fellowship of Surgeons occurred in 1540 with the grant of a charter to the Barber-Surgeons, effectively amalgamating the two bodies (Fig 1.8). The Charter is thought to have been arranged by Thomas Vicary, then Serjeant-Surgeon to The King and Master of the Barbers' Company. It provided a fee for the King and, of far more interest, provided the subject for a painting by Hans Holbein (Fig 1.9).

1.8 The Grace Cup

This cup was given to the Worshipful Company of Barber-Surgeons by Henry VIII in 1540. It was passed after Grace had been said at the end of the meal; after its passing, no more should be eaten until the following day. When Samuel Pepys dined in the 'Chyrurgeon's Hall' he recorded that 'we drunk the King's Health out of a gilt cup given by King Henry VIII to this company, with bells hanging at it, which every man is to ring by shaking after he hath drunk up the whole cup'.

(Courtesy Worshipful Company of Barbers)

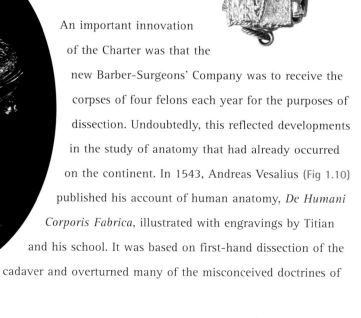

An important innovation of the Charter was that the new Barber-Surgeons' Company was to receive the corpses of four felons each year for the purposes of dissection. Undoubtedly, this reflected developments in the study of anatomy that had already occurred on the continent. In 1543, Andreas Vesalius (Fig 1.10) published his account of human anatomy, *De Humani Corporis Fabrica*, illustrated with engravings by Titian and his school. It was based on first-hand dissection of the cadaver and overturned many of the misconceived doctrines of

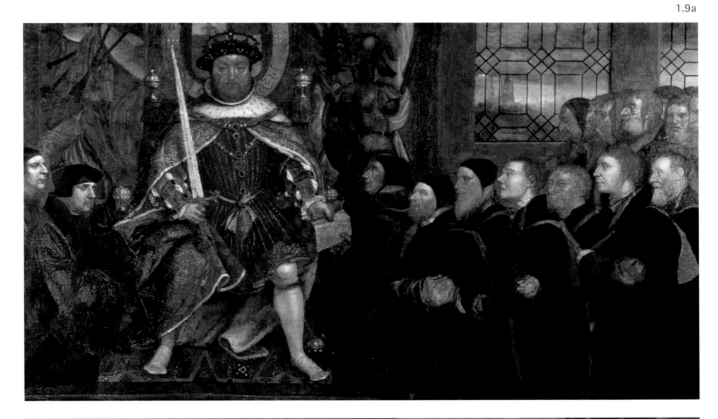

1.9a

1.9 King Henry VIII and the Barber-Surgeons

An X-ray examination by Professor Bertram Cohen revealed that the version now in the possession of the College (Fig 1.9a) might have been painted by Holbein's pupils over his original template, while Holbein's finished painting (Fig 1.9b) is preserved in Barbers' Hall. The College's version gives a glimpse, through a leaded window, of the old St Paul's Cathedral, subsequently destroyed in the Fire of London. Among the interesting portraits is that of John Chambre, the Reader in Anatomy of the Barber-Surgeons. He was brought in from the Royal College of Physicians and would have taught the traditional anatomy laid down by Galen.

In these paintings, Thomas Vicary is shown receiving the Charter from the King. Vicary (1490/1500–1562) was a surgeon in Maidstone in 1526 when Henry VIII required a dressing for the discharging sinus on his leg, now thought to have been chronic osteomyelitis dating from an injury sustained in a joust. The King approved of Vicary, and in 1528 made him Serjeant-Surgeon. The Company of Barbers elected Vicary Third Warden, and he became Master five times. It is believed that it was also Thomas Vicary who arranged the grant of a Charter to the Barber-Surgeons in 1540. Vicary was a survivor: he was still at court in the reign of Elizabeth I.

By Hans Holbein (1497–1543)

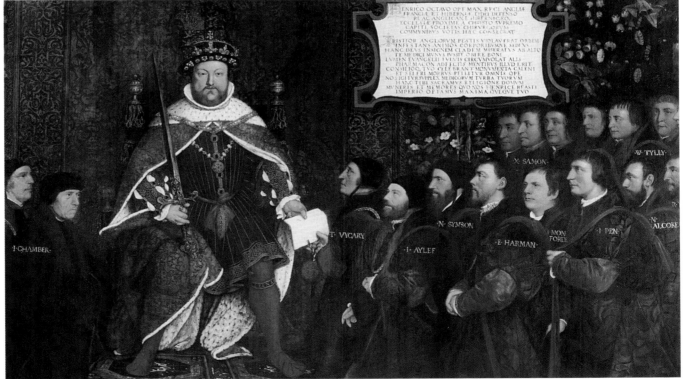

1.9b

1.10 Andreas Vesalius (1514–1564)

The key to the new anatomy was first-hand dissection of the cadaver. Each dissection became a voyage of discovery with the realisation that there was no single 'correct anatomy', but rather a whole spectrum of structures of the body. The modern reader who takes *Gray's Anatomy* for granted can hardly imagine how exciting Vesalius' publication must have been in the 16th century. For surgeons, it was as much a revolution as Tyndal's translation of the Bible had been for the person in the street, and, as with Tyndal's Bible, the invention of printing made it widely available and frequently copied.

*From De humani corporis fabrica libri septem.
Basileae (ex off Ioannis Oporini, 1543)*

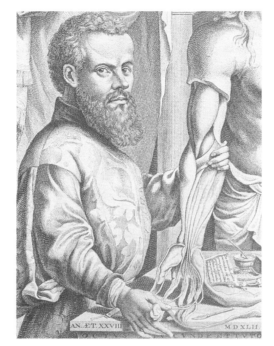

Galen. So exciting was the new anatomy that it became a subject for study by any reasonably educated gentleman, not only surgeons. Young surgeons were eager to see dissections, and the man who could teach anatomy from a dissected cadaver could command large fees (Fig 1.11).

In 1629 Charles I granted another charter (Fig 1.12) to the Barber-Surgeons' Company at the instigation of William Harvey (Figs 1.13 and 1.14), his Physician-in-Ordinary. This Charter ordered the surgeons to establish a Court of Examiners in Surgery that would, among other duties, certify ships' surgeons. The Court of Examiners effectively became the ruling body of the Fellowship (or Faculty, as it was sometimes known) of Surgeons within the Company.

1.11 Dissecting at Barber-Surgeons' Hall

John Bannister (1533–1610) is shown lecturing on anatomy at Barber-Surgeons' Hall in 1581. This painting, attributed to Nicholas Hilliard, is part of the collection of William Hunter now in Glasgow University Library.

(Courtesy Glasgow University Library)

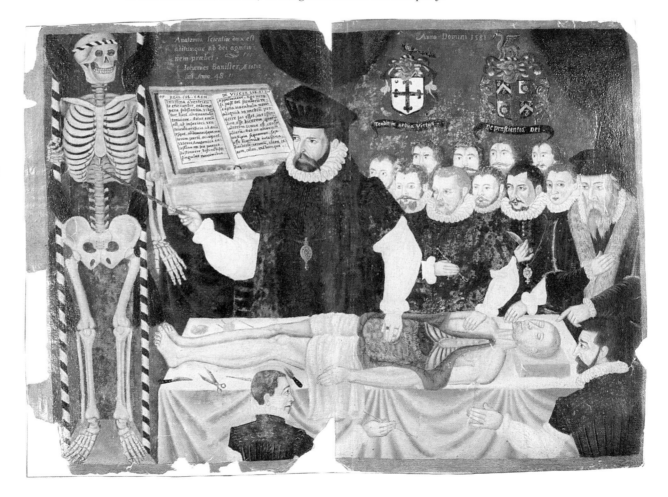

The importance of anatomy continued to grow. The Barber-Surgeons' Company wished to preserve their valuable monopoly, but lacked an appropriate place in which to study. In 1631 the Court of Examiners noted that 'the bodies have been a great annoyance to the tables, dresser boards and utensils in the upper kitchen by reason of the blood, filth and entrails of these anatomies and for the better accommodating of the anatomical affairs and preserving the kitchen to its own proper use', and accordingly decided to build a new anatomy theatre.

Inigo Jones designed an elaborate oval theatre, which opened in 1638.

For a considerable time there were few who could teach the new approaches to anatomy. The consequence was that many operations were still performed without correct knowledge of the underlying structures of the body. Nowhere was this more dangerous than in the ancient operation of lateral lithotomy, 'cutting for the stone' (Fig 1.15a–c).

By 1632 it was agreed that lectures on anatomy should be given by a surgeon of the Company rather than by a physician, as was the tradition. In 1646 Edward Arris left money to endow an anatomy demonstration, and his benefaction was emulated in 1655 by John Gale (the College commemorated both men in the Arris & Gale Lectureship). With the establishment of the Royal Navy in the second half of the 17th century, the Company's role in examining

1.12 The 1621 Charter of Charles I to the Barber-Surgeons' Company

In this Charter the Barber-Surgeons were ordered to set up a Court of Examiners that would, among other things, certify ships' surgeons.

(Courtesy Worshipful Company of Barbers)

1.13 William Harvey (1578–1657)

In 1600 Harvey went to Padua to study under Vesalius' pupil Fabricius ab Aquapendente, who had discovered the valves in peripheral veins, but still believed that blood ebbed and flowed. Harvey's experiments led him to an astoundingly imaginative jump: he postulated that there must exist tiny invisible channels in human tissues through which the blood would circulate. He published his discovery in 1628 and persuaded Charles I of its truth. To surgeons of his day, Harvey's ideas of the circulation of the blood were as esoteric as the minutiae of molecular biology are to many surgeons today. Many found it impossible to accept the concept of an invisible system of tiny blood vessels. Indeed, such vessels were not seen until 1649 when Henry Power of Cambridge found them in a frog's lung, using a simple microscope.

Plaster cast of a bust by Peter Scheemaker
(original now in The Royal College of Physicians)

1.13

1.14 Illustration from the first edition of Harvey's treatise on blood circulation

From Exercitatio anatomica de motu cordis et sanguinis in animalibus.
Francofurti, sumpt. Guilielmi Fitzeri, 1628

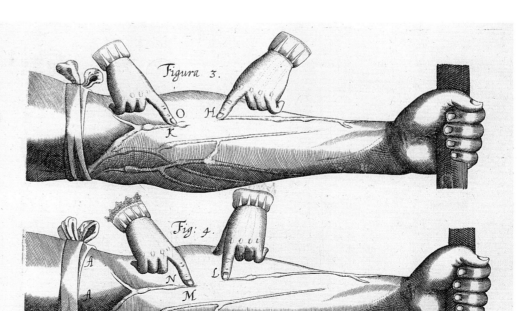

1.15a–c Lithotomy operation

Lithotomy was a notoriously dangerous operation
(Fig 1.16a). As there exists only a narrow gap between
the superficial and transverse perineal arteries,
making the incision half an inch too far on either
side risks uncontrollable haemorrhage in the depths
of the wound. One in three patients did not survive.
One who did survive was Samuel Pepys (Fig 1.16b),
who had a bladder stone the size of a tennis ball
removed on 26 March 1659 by Thomas Hollyer
(1609–1690) (Fig 1.16c), a surgeon and lithotomist
at St Thomas's and St Bartholomew's hospitals and
a contemporary of Harvey. Pepys was number 31 in
Hollyer's series for that year: numbers 32 through
35 all died. Pepys remained
Hollyer's good friend and
celebrated 26 March with
a feast for the rest of his
life. High mortality from the
operation continued until
William Cheselden worked out
the anatomy of the perineum.

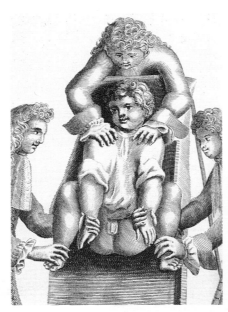

1.15a Drawing from Tolet, F., *Treatise on Lithotomy*, 1682

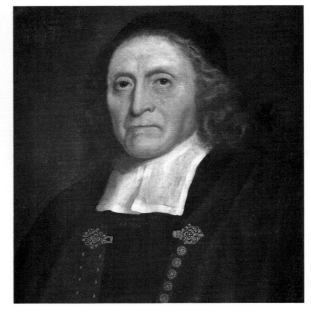

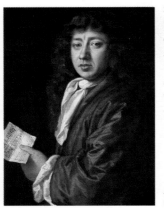

1.15b Portrait of Samuel Pepys by
John Hayls, 1666 (Courtesy National
Portrait Gallery, London)

1.15c Portrait of Thomas Hollyer by an anonymous artist

1.16 Richard Wiseman (1620–1676)

Wiseman was apprenticed to Richard Smith in the
Barber-Surgeons' Company in 1637. During the
Civil War, he served in the West Country and saw
many gunshot wound treatments, making careful
notes of their outcome. After the rout at Truro,
he escaped with the Prince of Wales to France in
1645 and returned with him to Scotland in 1650.
When the Scottish army was defeated at the
Battle of Worcester in 1651, Wiseman was
captured and imprisoned in Chester, where he
continued to treat the sick and wounded. He was
released in 1652 and went to London, became a
Freeman of the Barber-Surgeons' Company, and
set up in practice in the Old Bailey. An unrepentant
Royalist, he was accused of helping James Read
escape from the Tower of London and was himself
imprisoned for a second time. On being set free,
he joined the Spanish Navy and served in the
West Indies, where he is thought to have
contracted tuberculosis. He rejoined Charles II on
his Restoration in 1660 and was made Surgeon-
in-Ordinary. He wrote up some 660 of his cases
in *Severall Chirugicall Treatises*, which became
the standard textbook of the time, largely because
of its excellent English prose that attracted the
praise even of Samuel Johnson. It included
descriptions of operations for aneurysm.

ships' surgeons gained importance and, indeed, the position of naval surgeon was crucial in the
development of many surgeons' careers at that time, including Richard Wiseman, sometimes
called the 'Father of English Surgery' (Fig 1.16).

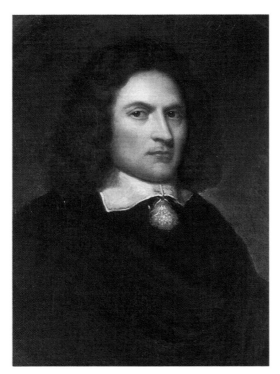

Anonymous

By the mid-18th century, a new breed of surgeon had
appeared on the scene, experienced in the hard school
of military surgery in a succession of continental
wars and with a better knowledge of anatomy.
The Faculty of Surgeons was no longer a small and
insignificant group: they were clever, educated, rich
and increasingly powerful. Its members began to find
the rules of the Barber-Surgeons' Company irksome
and sought independence from them. The surgeons
of London were not by any means the first to seek
separation of their profession from the craft of the
barbers: it had been achieved in Edinburgh in 1718, in
Berlin in 1725, and in Paris by 1743. Two men were
responsible for the separation in London: John Ranby
and William Cheselden (Fig 1.17).

1.17 William Cheselden (1688–1752)

Cheselden was famous as an anatomist and operative surgeon. By 1711 he was a leading teacher of the new anatomy and had written a best-selling textbook. Then he overstepped the mark: Cheselden began to teach by dissection away from Barber-Surgeons' Hall. When the Master admonished him, he went to Amsterdam where he learned the technique of lateral lithotomy. On returning to London Cheselden studied the operation further and worked out how it could be done more safely, even if it meant enlarging the wound to control bleeding from a deep vessel. He taught the improved technique with great generosity. Towards the end of his career Cheselden reported only three deaths in his last 50 patients, a mortality rate unmatched even a century later in the general hospitals of London. He was also the first to perform iridectomy.

Upon his retirement in 1737, Cheselden lived in the Royal Hospital, Chelsea, and joined the Court of Assistants of the Company of Barber-Surgeons as a Warden. He was instrumental in bringing about the separation of the surgeons from the barbers, and succeeded John Ranby as Master of the Company of Surgeons in 1746.

By Jonathan Richardson

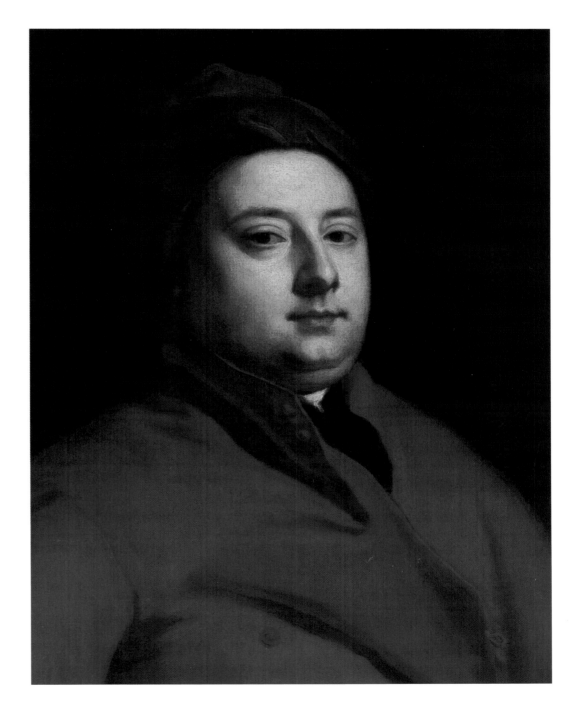

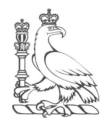

CHAPTER 2

The Company *of* Surgeons

2.1 The Ranby Cup

This cup, a gift to the College by John Ranby, was made by Eliza Godfrey in 1745. The inscription reads *'Die Julij primo MDCCXLV hoc qualecumque suae in Fratres Observantiae Monumentum Dignissimae Chirurgorum Londinensium Societati Consecrat Joannes Ranby'* (First July 1745 John Ranby consecrates this trifle as a memorial of his regard for his brethren to the Worshipful Company of Surgeons of London).

John Ranby (1703–1773) 'qualified', ie was made Free of the Company, at the age of 19, became a Fellow of the Royal Society and was a trusted friend of the monarch. In 1737, he looked after Queen Caroline during her last illness, a strangulated umbilical hernia, which he incised with a predictably fatal result. He became Serjeant-Surgeon in 1740 and accompanied George II to the Battle of Dettingen. There he treated William, Duke of Cumberland, who had received a musket ball through the leg.

Unfortunately, no likeness of Ranby has survived.

2.2 Unofficial coat of arms adopted by the Surgeons' Company

The coat of arms includes two figures representing Machaon and Podalirius, the sons of Aesculapius, the Greek god of medicine. One is holding a surgeon's knife, the other a broken arrow, a symbol of healing. Motto: *Quae prosunt omnibus artes* (The arts that are of service to all).

Negotiations to separate the surgeons from the barbers within the Company of Barber-Surgeons began in 1744. The surgeons submitted a petition to Parliament to set up a committee. The chairman of the committee was William Cheselden's son-in-law, a physician named Charles Cotes, and Cheselden paid £550 of his own money to smooth the passage of the Bill. The barbers submitted a counter-petition, but by May 1745 the Bill had received Royal Assent and the Company of Surgeons came into being. Full of enthusiasm, the Court of Assistants of the new Company met in Stationers' Hall on 1 July 1745. John Ranby celebrated the occasion with the gift of a handsome silver cup (Fig 2.1) and took the oath twice, first as Freeman of the Company and second as its first Master.

Under the terms of the Act of 1745, the Barbers retained all the corporate property of the Company of Barber-Surgeons, save the bequests of Edward Arris and John Gale for anatomy lectures. The surgeons were incorporated under the name of 'The Master, Governors and Commonalty of the Art and Science of Surgeons of London'. They established a governing body, the Court of Assistants, 21 of whom were appointed for life. From the Court of Assistants, a master and two wardens were elected annually, as well as a court of ten examiners, who were also appointed for life.

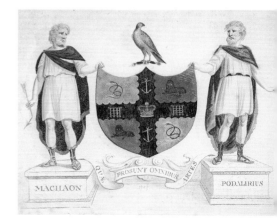

2.2

The new Company needed a new coat of arms but rather than seek an expensive patent from the College of Heralds, they hired a jobbing painter named Brookshead to paint them an unofficial one for three guineas. It is these unofficial arms (Fig 2.2) that appear on the cup Ranby gave to the College.

The Freemen of the Company were to enjoy the same surgical privileges as the surgeons of the old Barber-Surgeons' Company. They continued, under the Act of Union and Charter of Charles I 'to oversee, rule and leet offices', including service on juries. An important additional duty of the new Company of Surgeons, in keeping with their long-standing responsibility for the navy, was to examine surgeons' mates for the army (Fig 2.3).

2.3a

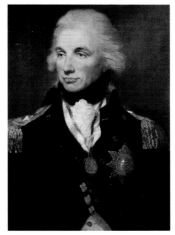
2.3b

The Worshipful Company of Barbers continued to bear its 1569 coat of arms, retained ownership of Barber-Surgeons' Hall in Monkwell Square, and remains to this day – along with 99 other livery companies – an important part of the history and fabric of the City of London. Today its principal concerns are its charities, among which is The Royal College of Surgeons of England.

2.3 Medical board record

The Company and the country's armed forces had a close relationship stemming from the examination of naval and army surgeons, as well as the assessment by the Company of claims for compensation for injuries incurred on active duty.

A particularly interesting entry in the Court of Examiner's minute book (Fig 2.3a) records the medical examination of Rear Admiral Sir Horatio Nelson on 12 October 1797. The Court valued the injury he had received at the Seige of Calvi in July 1794 as equal to the loss of an eye. Nelson (Fig 2.3b) was back before the Court the following year, after losing his right arm at Santa Cruz. Throughout that autumn he had to report regularly on the continuing discharge from the sinus in the amputation stump, which only ceased when the ligature 'attended by evil odours fell into the dressing like a spent snake, to trouble no more'.

Portrait of Lord Nelson by Lemuel Francis Abbott, 1797
(Courtesy National Portrait Gallery, London)

In 1745 only about 90 surgeons practised in London, but from the outset this relatively small number distinguished themselves from general practitioners. The Court of Assistants drew up bylaws that included bans on concomitant practice as an apothecary or in midwifery; this put the control of the new Company firmly in the hands of hospital surgeons rather than the general practitioners. The period of apprenticeship was set at seven years. The fee or 'consideration' paid by an apprentice to his master varied but could be as high as £500, worth perhaps 100 times as much today. These fees were an important source of income for senior surgeons.

'Freedom', or qualification, depended on satisfying the Court of Examiners in a test that covered knowledge of Latin as well as medical topics. In practice, the Court seldom insisted on the full period of seven years' service; nevertheless, many surgeons found it easier to join the army or the navy for a short time and then retire to set up practice outside London where they would be free of the control of the Company.

2.4

2.4 Surgeons' Hall

The Hall was built next to Newgate Prison on the site of today's Central Criminal Court in the Old Bailey. William Cheselden, a talented amateur architect, drew up plans, but they were rejected. Further designs were commissioned from William Kent (1684–1748) and George Dance the Elder (1700–1768), but these were deemed too costly. In the end, the architect selected was William Jones (d. 1757), who also designed the Rotunda at Ranelagh. It is Jones' building that appears in this engraving by Benjamin Cole.

The most urgent task of the new Company was to teach anatomy. They chose for their new hall a site in the Old Bailey next to Newgate Prison (Fig 2.4) and began to pull down the existing houses in 1747.

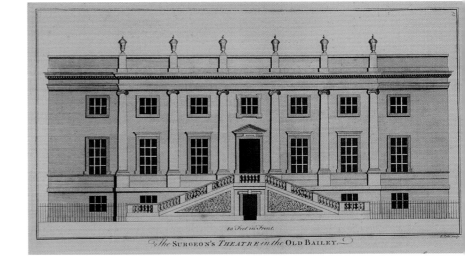

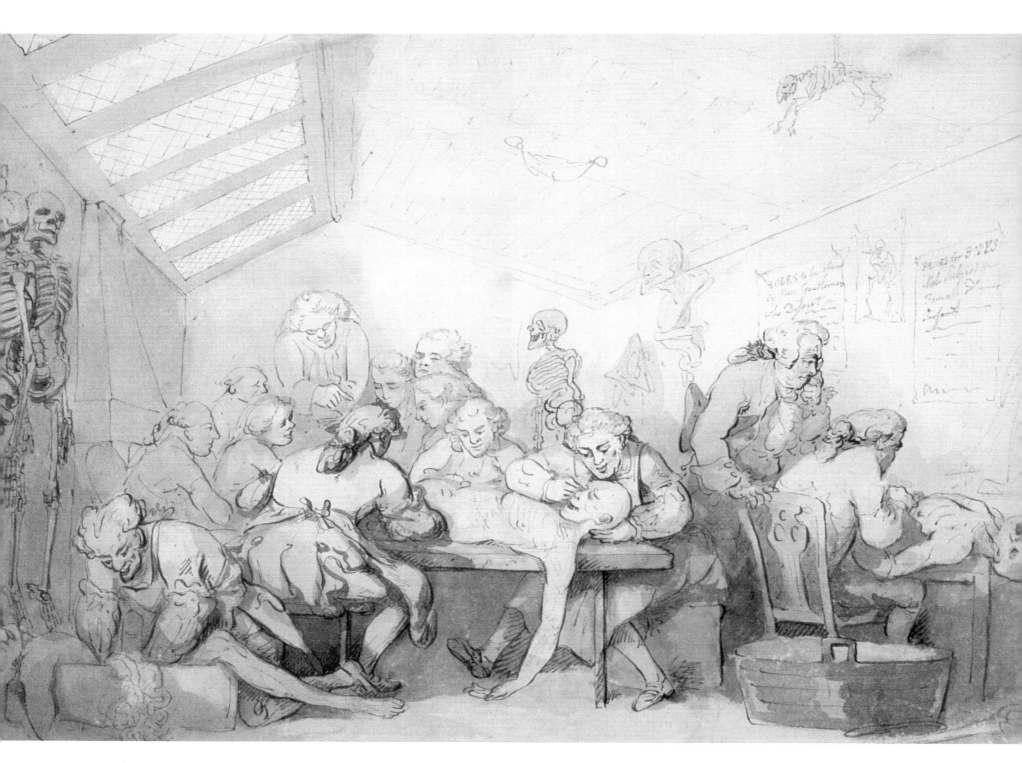

2.5 The Dissecting Room

Rowlandson was a friend of the Hunters. This painting shows William Hunter standing on the left, with Matthew Baillie on his right and John Hunter on his left.

By Thomas Rowlandson (1756–1827)

The first part to be built was the anatomy theatre. After seemingly endless delays as one design after another was rejected, plans by William Jones were accepted. This hiatus was nearly the undoing of the new Company: for almost a decade, anatomy lectures were suspended for lack of a suitable theatre. The Company rescinded the existing rule that dissections and demonstrations of anatomy could only be performed at Surgeons' Hall.

For practical purposes, the management of the Company was in the hands of the Court of Examiners. From 1748 onwards, the Court of Examiners only convened a meeting of the full Court of Assistants when they deemed it necessary. Older members who were outside this clique regretted the good old days, for the new Company had neither social nor charitable activities, and the teaching of anatomy had come to a halt. This was especially unfortunate because the hiatus came just when there was a major change in the methods of teaching anatomy: students in Paris, instead of listening to the professor while a demonstrator pointed out the relevant parts of the dissection, were performing the dissection themselves (Fig 2.5).

2.6a

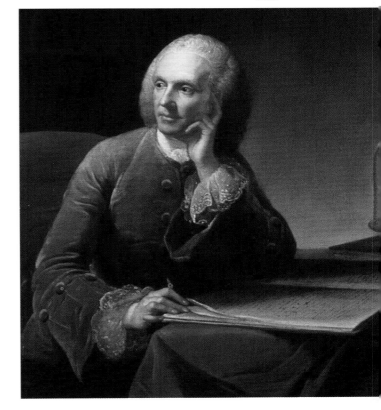

The teaching vacuum was filled by a growing number of private schools of anatomy outside the aegis of the Company, similar to those of William Cheselden a generation before. One of the most important was in Great Windmill Street in Soho. It was run by a young Scotsman named William Hunter (Fig 2.6). The Windmill Street School was not merely a lucrative business, it was also a centre for the serious scientific study of physiology and anatomy. From Hunter and his pupils came many important and original observations. By 1748, William Hunter's school was already so successful that he sent for his younger brother John to help him prepare specimens and teach pupils. John Hunter went on to become a skilled anatomist and surgeon,

2.6 William Hunter (1718–1783)

William Hunter obtained the Grand Diploma of the Company in 1749 (Fig 2.6b) and his medical degree from Glasgow in 1750. He established his extremely successful private school in Covent Garden before moving it to Great Windmill Street (Fig 2.6c). Like other anatomists, he was supplied with cadavers by the so-called 'Resurrection Men'. He left the Company, attained the licence of the Royal College of Physicians in 1756 and became obstetrician to Queen Charlotte in 1762. He was the first Professor of Anatomy at the Royal Academy in 1768.

Portrait of Hunter by Robert Edge Pine

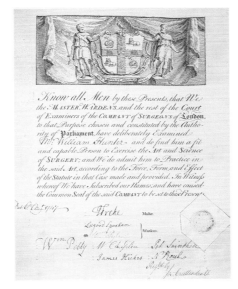

2.6b

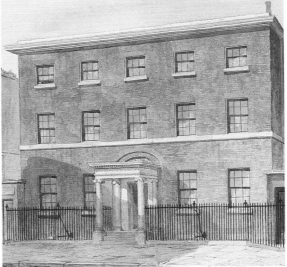

2.6c

and his research into the form and structure of living things made him an important pioneer in the scientific aspects of surgery. The younger Hunter served on the Court of Assistants of the Company, but played little part in its work. He did, however, have an enormous impact on the subsequent history of the Company through the legacy of his collection of comparative anatomy and pathology (Fig 2.7, overleaf).

John Hunter

John Hunter was considered a dull scholar who often played truant. It seems likely that he was dyslexic, a condition that might have contributed to his being less interested in reading and more interested in experimenting. Throughout his life Hunter was good with his hands, whether dissecting or operating, and he possessed an uncommon ability to recognise patterns in things. His preference for trying things out for himself rather than reading about the works of others gave him an original perspective, unhampered by conventional wisdom.

John Hunter spent his first 12 years in London dissecting and undertaking experiments in his brother William's anatomy school. A three-year commission in the army during the War of the Spanish Succession offered him an opportunity to expand his surgical knowledge for the first time without his brother's guidance, and to indulge his passion for natural history and collection of specimens. Throughout the siege of Belle Isle and the successful campaign in Portugal, experience with gunshot wounds taught Hunter that it was unnecessary either to cauterise them or to extract musket balls that were doing no harm. Because he seldom read the literature, he was unaware that these lessons had been propounded by Ambroise Paré a century before.

John Hunter returned from the army to set up in practice in London, where he continued collecting, studying, dissecting and undertaking experiments. He was a pioneer in applying the experimental approach to the study of the structure and function of living matter. To support his research, he collected specimens of human and animal anatomy and pathology for comparative purposes. Hunter had a wide circle of friends and colleagues – including other scientists, artists and explorers such as Sir Joseph Banks, George Stubbs and Daniel Solander – many of whom brought back specimens from their voyages or recorded examples of new species seen in menageries or travelling shows.

In addition to blood-letting much of the surgeon's everyday practice consisted of inoculation with matter from a smallpox vesicle, which conferred protection but sometimes led to full-blown smallpox. Hunter's friend and former pupil, Edward Jenner, had noticed that milkmaids in his Gloucestershire village who caught the lesser disease cowpox in the course of their occupation escaped smallpox when an epidemic spread to their village. In a letter to Hunter in 1796, Jenner wondered whether the one might confer protection from the other. Hunter told him to stop thinking and try the experiment.

2.7 John Hunter (1728–1793)

By Sir Joshua Reynolds (1723–1792)

2.7a John Hunter's tankard

This tankard, made in 1730, is engraved with the arms of the Hunter family. It was given to the College by Hunter's nephew, Captain Everard Home, in 1869. The elaborate embossed decoration was added later.

2.7a

2.7b

In this letter, Hunter urged Edward Jenner to try the cowpox experiment. Jenner was one of Hunter's pupils and close friends.

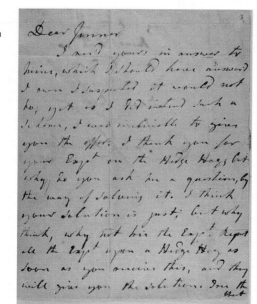

2.7c Indian Rhinoceros

A young male rhinoceros arrived in London in 1790 and was put on show at Clark's exhibition of curiosities at the Exeter 'Change & Lyceum' in the Strand. It died in Portsmouth in 1793 after damaging a leg while on tour around the country.

Painting believed to have been commissioned from George Stubbs (1724–1800) by John Hunter

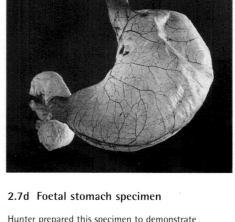

2.7d

2.7c

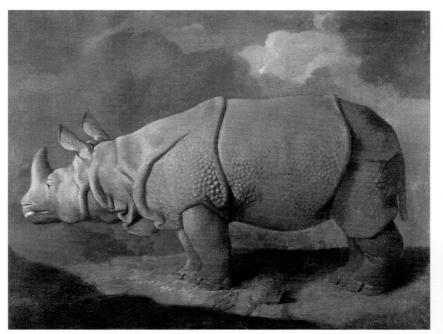

2.7d Foetal stomach specimen

Hunter prepared this specimen to demonstrate the circulation in a human foetal stomach. It is an excellent example of Hunter's technical skills. He injected the arteries with a red dye and preserved the specimen in oil of turpentine, rather than the customary alcohol, to prevent the tissues from becomimg opaque.

Photograph by Elaine Duigenan

2.7e Cherokee Indian

This portrait, together with a companion portrait of another young Cherokee man, is believed to have been commissioned by John Hunter. These two Native Americans fought on the British side during the War of American Independence. When they came to England in 1790-91, they were treated as celebrities in London society.

By William Hodges (1744–1797)

2.7f A Malay Lady

According to William Clift, this girl was sent to be educated in England, where she became a patient of John Hunter. This portrait was painted by Hunter's brother-in-law some time between 1780 and 1788. The subject died of a psoas abscess.

By Robert Home (1752–1834)

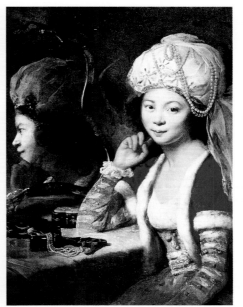

2.7f

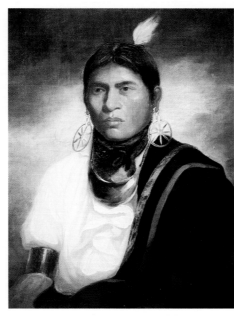

2.7e

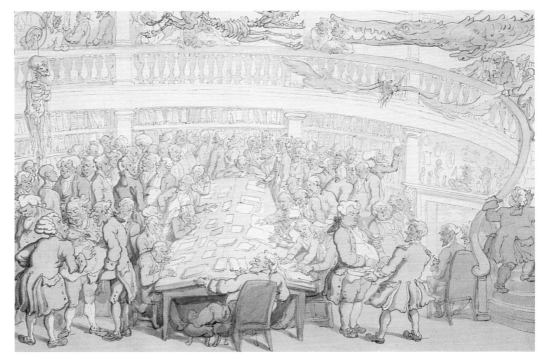

2.8

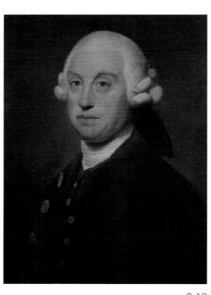

2.9

2.10

2.8 John Heaviside lecturing at Surgeons' Hall

By Thomas Rowlandson (1756–1827)

2.9 Sir Caesar Hawkins (1711–1786)

Hawkins served on the Court of Examiners for 31 years. He was much in demand as a surgeon, became Serjeant-Surgeon to both George II and George III, and was the first surgeon to be made a baronet. He seems to have made a living mainly from blood-letting, though he obviously practised lithotomy, as a cutting gorget is named after him.

By William Hogarth (1697–1764)

2.10 Percivall Pott (1713–1788)

Pott was famous in his day for his teaching at St Bartholomew's Hospital. His many writings, all clearly expressed, covered a wide range of topics from fistula-in-ano to hernia and curvature of the spine. He served on the Court of Examiners for 29 years and was Master in 1765.

By George Romney (1734–1802)

William Hunter was appointed Master of Anatomy by the Company in 1753, but there were no prosected specimens with which to teach. Moreover, although from time to time the Company appointed other eminent Professors of Anatomy – including William Blizard, John Abernethy and Astley Cooper – no regular system of lectures was established (Fig 2.8). William Hunter finally left the Company to take up gynaecology and obstetrics, joined the Royal College of Physicians and eventually became Physician Extraordinary to The Queen.

The Company of Surgeons was in effect run by the Court of Examiners. These ten senior surgeons (Figs 2.9 and 2.10) met monthly to examine naval and army surgeons. In times of war they were very busy, seeing as many as 50 candidates at a time. Sir Zachary Cope summarises the state of affairs at this time: 'The Company dragged on its uninspired existence without more than an occasional criticism or attempt at improvement until 1789–90, when John Gunning was Master'. Gunning rebuked the Court of Assistants in his celebrated 'Phillipic' of 1790:

> Your theatre is without lectures, your library without books is converted into an office for your clerk and your committee room has become an eating parlour... I am sorry to observe that you have instituted lectures neither in surgery nor indeed in anatomy of any degree of importance.

It was time for change, and the catalyst was John Hunter. When he died in 1793, Hunter left his enormous collection of some 14,000 specimens, dissections and notes in the trust of his executors – his brother-in-law Everard Home and nephew Matthew Baillie (Fig 2.11) – with the instructions that it be offered for sale to the government. It was this gesture that led to long-awaited reforms and the transformation of the Company into a College.

Hunter's executors petitioned Parliament to purchase the collection, and in 1799 the Treasury agreed, with a grant of £15,000 (worth perhaps £300,000 today). Hunter's collection was transferred to the Company in a Treasury Minute, with an accompanying stipulation that the Surgeons' Company build a museum to house the collection, and that it be governed by a board of trustees.

The Court of Examiners had already decided to sell Surgeons' Hall in the Old Bailey and buy the property at 41 Lincoln's Inn Fields; the Court of Assistants was informed of the decision on 19 May 1796. Having agreed to the purchase, however, the Company found that under the Act of 1745, they were not permitted to hold lands, tenements or rents exceeding the value of £200 per annum, and the houses in Lincoln's Inn Fields had cost £5,500. To circumvent the Act, the houses were conveyed in the names of the Master and Wardens as trustees, a decision that was to assume great importance a few years later. The Company took possession on 5 January 1797.

With the move to Lincoln's Inn Fields came the suggestion that the by-laws be brought up-to-date. Among the proposed changes were that the name of the Company should be changed to 'College', and the Master and Wardens to 'President' and 'Vice-Presidents'. These proposals reflected the aspirations of the Fellows: the change from a 'Company', with its overtones of a trade guild, to a 'College', with its implication of an academic discipline to be taught, learned and examined. The consent of George III was obtained for the use of the word 'Royal'.

2.11 Matthew Baillie (1761–1823)

Baillie was a pioneering figure in the discipline of morbid anatomy. The Royal College of Physicians presented the College with 1,251 preparations that he had made, but all were destroyed by the bombing during the Second World War.

By Joseph Nollekens (1734–1823), 1812

A bill incorporating these proposals was hastened through the House of Commons and sent to the House of Lords in April 1797, where it was held up. Two of their Lordships lived in Lincoln's Inn Fields and did not fancy having surgeons as their neighbours, and there was the technical problem of transporting the bodies of felons from the gallows to Lincoln's Inn Fields. In addition, the Members of the Company felt aggrieved because they had not been consulted. In response to these concerns, the Court of Assistants agreed to buy premises nearer Newgate, but this and other attempts at compromise were unsuccessful.

James Earle was Master of the Company in 1798 and Serjeant-Surgeon to George III. He suggested that it might be possible to obtain a Charter directly from the Crown. A Royal Charter, however, could not supersede an Act of Parliament unless that Act had been rendered invalid by some irregularity. Vicary Gibbs presented the argument for invalidity by demonstrating that the Court of Examiners had acted irregularly in 1796 in selling the old building without the sanction of the Court of Assistants. The Company was ipso facto dissolved.

Another two years passed before the Charter establishing the College gained approval by the law officers of the Crown. The Great Seal was affixed on 22 March 1800.

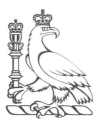

CHAPTER 3

The Early Years
of the College

3.1 The Beadle's staff

Now known colloquially as the 'travelling mace', the staff is engraved with the coat of arms of the Company and inscribed 'The Royal College of Surgeons in London 22nd March 1800'. It was made in 1803 of silver on an ebony staff 5ft 8in long.

The first meeting of the Court of Assistants of the new Royal College of Surgeons in London was held on 10 April 1800 (Fig 3.1). All Members of the former Company were invited to join the new body as Members of the Royal College of Surgeons (MRCS). More than 1,000 accepted, though it took one Member more than 40 years to make up his mind (Fig 3.2).

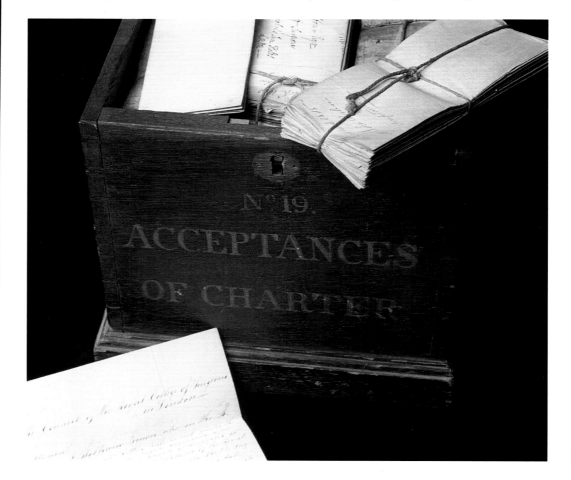

3.2 Acceptances box

All of the Members of the Company of Surgeons had to submit their assent to the new Charter. This box contains all the acceptances.

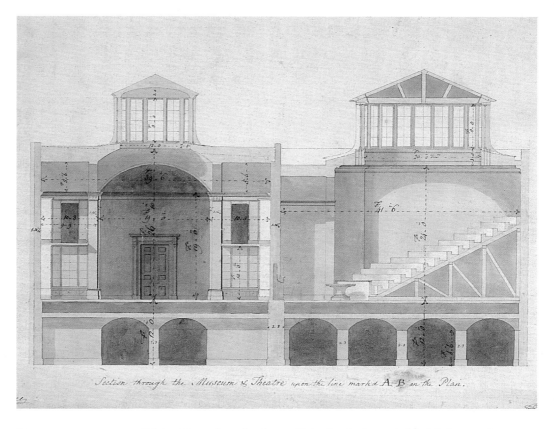

3.3 Designs for the new College

One of the design drawings by George Dance the Younger (1741–1825) and James Lewis, showing a section through the museum and theatre.

Section through the Museum & Theatre upon the line marked A. B on the Plan.

To act as conservator of John Hunter's collection, still in Castle Street behind Leicester Square, the Court appointed William Clift, Hunter's assistant from 1792. The building at 42 Lincoln's Inn Fields became vacant and was bought in 1802 to move the collection closer to the College. The decision to purchase the building was once again made by the Court of Examiners acting ultra vires, not the Court of Assistants; moreover, they failed to notify the newly appointed Hunterian Trustees.

Plans for a new building on the Lincoln's Inn Fields site were drawn up by George Dance the Younger and James Lewis (Fig 3.3), but the costs were too high. The College decided to approach the government for assistance; thanks to Lord Grenville's support (Fig 3.4), Parliament granted £15,000 towards the cost of the building. Work started in 1805.

In 1810 a third tranche of money was approved by Parliament, bringing the total government grants to purchase property and build a new College accommodating the Hunterian Collection to £42,000. This building was finished in 1813 and had a grand porticoed entrance in Lincoln's Inn Fields for those on the Courts of Examiners and Assistants (Fig 3.5); Members, however, had to use the back door in Portugal Street, an affront that rankled for years.

3.4 Lord Grenville (1759–1834)

After the death of John Hunter, Lord Grenville was instrumental in allocating funds so that the College could obtain the Hunterian Collection. He was Foreign Secretary (1791–1801) at the start of the Napoleonic Wars, and Prime Minister when the French invasion fleet was mustering at Boulogne. Grenville was later head of the Ministry of 'All the Talents' which abolished the slave trade.

By Thomas Phillips, 1810

3.5 View of the new College from
Walk Through London

By Edward Pugh, 1817

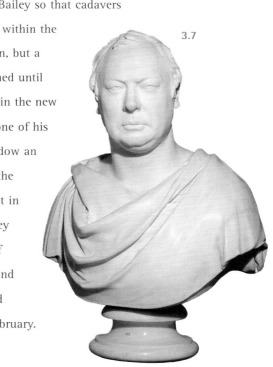

3.6 Sir William Blizard (1743–1835)

Blizard was a pupil of Percivall Pott and teacher of John Abernethy. In 1785 he received permission from The London Hospital to deliver lectures on anatomy and surgery in rooms in the hospital, thus founding the London Hospital Medical College, the first medical school to be connected with a hospital. In 1791 he founded the Samaritan Society of The London Hospital to assist patients after they left the hospital. He was Master of the College in 1814, President in 1822–23 and the founder and first President of the Hunterian Society. He retired from the Court of Examiners at the age of 92.

By John Opie (1761–1807)

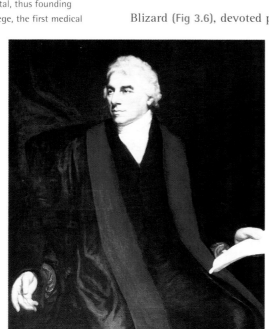

3.7 Sir Everard Home (1756–1832)

Although he was the executor and brother-in-law of John Hunter, this did not stop Home from destroying many of Hunter's records after trying to pass them off as his own work. Paradoxically, Home was the prime mover in obtaining the Hunterian Collection for the College.

By Joseph Nollekens (1737–1823)

Members of the Court added many of their own specimens to Hunter's collection. Sir William Blizard (Fig 3.6), devoted pupil and admirer of John Hunter, provided 900 of his own preparations, which included 'some of the best injections of the absorbents (lymphatics) in London effected by his own hands'.

The new Royal College still did little by way of offering instruction. A warehouse was hired near the Old Bailey so that cadavers of executed felons could be dissected within the statutory 400 yards of Newgate Prison, but a proper course of lectures was postponed until an appropriate theatre could be built in the new building. In 1800 Blizard persuaded one of his former pupils, Samuel Jackson, to endow an annual prize of £10 to the author of the best dissertation on a practical subject in surgery. Since then, winning the Jacksonian Prize has been the key note of many eminent surgical careers. In 1813, at the opening of the new building, Sir Everard Home (Fig 3.7) announced that he and Matthew Baillie, John Hunter's nephew and other executor, would endow an annual oration to be given on Hunter's birthday, 14 February. Home gave the inaugural oration in 1814.

3.7

Other changes followed. The *Apothecaries Act* of 1815 provided that general practitioners in England and Wales would be allowed to practise only if they had undergone an approved five-year apprenticeship and passed the examination of the Society of Apothecaries. Three times the College tried to resist this advance, although time has shown it to be an important measure in establishing medicine as a profession in Britain.

To no avail, the College put forward its own bill to regulate all those practising surgery. Next, the College tried to gain control of surgery in the whole of Great Britain and Ireland; this was overcome by objections from the older established colleges in Ireland and Scotland. Finally, the College proposed reforms to its Royal Charter, including mandatory attendance on the practice of a hospital in addition to six years of apprenticeship. This was the College's first effort to set standards in surgical education.

In 1822 these changes to the Charter were approved by the King. The Master and Wardens were henceforth to be known as President and Vice-Presidents, and the Court of Assistants became the Council. The Court of Examiners retained its old name. Sir Everard Home, the inaugural President, persuaded George IV to visit the College. On this occasion the King presented a splendid mace (Fig 3.8), and later the same year granted the College an official coat of arms (Fig 3.9).

Over the next few years, the College continued trying to extend its authority beyond London. It met considerable opposition, especially from those practising and teaching surgery in towns other than those the College recognised (Dublin, Edinburgh, Glasgow and Aberdeen), for there were already strong surgical traditions in towns such as Norwich, and new ones were springing up in centres like Leeds and Liverpool.

Meanwhile, the College's governance was being challenged by its Members, led by Thomas Wakley, founder and editor of the *Lancet* (Fig 3.10). He was at first aided and abetted by William Lawrence of

3.8 College mace presented by George IV in 1822

Made by Rundell, Bridge and Rundell in 1822, the mace is of silver gilt. It is 4ft 4in in length and weighs 14lb 9oz. It still bears the old (unofficial) arms of the Company and is inscribed '*Ex munificentia Augustissimi Monarchae George IV De Gra: Brittaniarum Regis &c Collegii Regalis Chirurgorum Patroni Optimi An.Dom. MDCCCXXII Everardo Home, Baronetto, Primo Praeside*'.

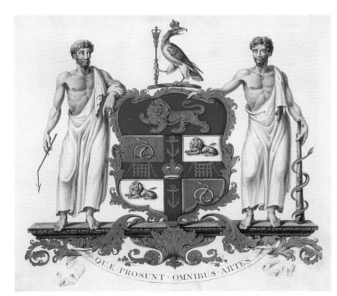

3.9 The official coat of arms of 1822

3.10 Thomas Wakley (1795–1862)

The 'battling surgeon', founding editor of the *Lancet*, Wakley was a ceaseless reformer who tried to improve the management of the College. He was later famous for his successful campaign against flogging in the army.

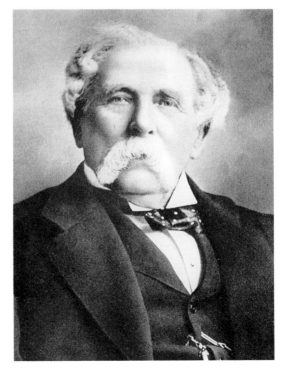

3.8

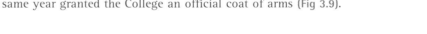

3.10

3.11 Sir William Lawrence (1783–1867)

Lawrence had been Abernethy's apprentice and was a fierce supporter of Wakley until he was elected to Council, whereupon he became decidedly more conservative. He served on Council from 1825 until his death and was President twice, in 1846 and 1855. He had a long career as a surgeon and lecturer on surgery at St Bartholomew's Hospital, and indeed was one of the most noted medical lecturers of his time. He was on his way upstairs to administer an examination when he suffered a fatal stroke.

By Charles Turner

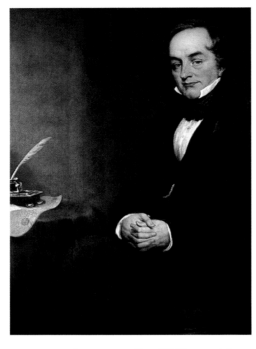

3.12 John Abernethy (1764–1831)

Pupil of John Hunter and William Blizard, Abernethy was elected to St Bartholomew's Hospital in 1787 at the age of 23 and established the medical school there, where his lectures were very popular. He became a Fellow of the Royal Society in 1796. He was celebrated for developing John Hunter's operation for aneurysm. Abernethy was President in the midst of Thomas Wakley's attacks on the College in 1826.

By Charles William Pegler

3.13 Notice dated 10 March 1831

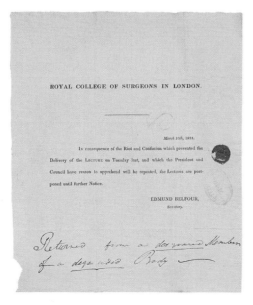

St Bartholomew's Hospital (Fig 3.11). They attacked the College for its archaic system of life tenure on Council and pressed for representation for general surgical practitioners who were not on the staff of the great London hospitals. At a public meeting, the rebels resolved to petition Parliament, which had spent so much taxpayers' money on the Hunterian Collection and the College buildings, to enquire into the governance of the College.

The President at this time, John Abernethy (Fig 3.12), called two extraordinary meetings of Council, but they resolved nothing. Then came a memorandum supporting Wakley and Lawrence signed by the most eminent of the younger consultants in the teaching hospitals of London (most of whom, incidentally, later became Presidents of the College). Abernethy warned his Council that it would be impolitic to ignore the protesters, but they did.

Nevertheless, Wakley achieved one of his objectives when, in 1827, Parliament demanded to know how its money had been spent and asked for details of the management of College affairs, the hours the library and museum were open, how many candidates took the examinations, and what proportion of them passed. These questions were all highly embarrassing.

Lawrence was elected to Council in 1828, leaving Wakley to continue his attacks alone. Wakley caused a scene during the Hunterian

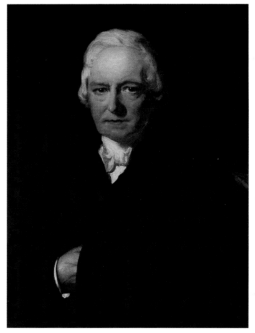

3.12

Oration in February 1831, but it came to nothing. He did the same at the next College lecture in March (Fig 3.13): Wakley burst in with 400 Members from London and the suburbs. When the President and Council arrived, they were guarded by a team of Bow Street runners. An angry hubbub ensued in which Wakley was seized by the collar and struck on the shoulder by the truncheon of Constable Leadbitter. Half a dozen others were also injured. Eventually the crowd moved off to Bow Street, where Wakley charged his assailant before the Chief Magistrate. In the end, neither Wakley nor the College pressed charges.

3.14 The Resurrectionists

It was public concern over the activities of the Resurrection Men (people who dug up cadavers from graveyards and supplied them to others for anatomical studies) that led to the *Anatomy Act* of 1832. The Act made available to the medical schools a legitimate supply of cadavers from the deceased paupers from the workhouses. This practice was one of the chief causes of the public's dread of the workhouse in the 19th century.

By Thomas Rowlandson (1756-1827)

At the same time, a grisly scandal erupted. The famous private anatomy schools, including that of the Hunters, had long been supplied with cadavers by the so-called 'Resurrection Men' (Fig 3.14). To satisfy the increasing demand for cadavers, some of the more enterprising resurrectionists decided to anticipate nature: two were found guilty of murder in Edinburgh in 1828, and three years later two more were convicted of the same crime in London (Fig 3.15). One of their victims had been taken to the King's College Hospital, then in Portugal Street, a stone's throw from the College. The Court of Examiners hastily drew up recommendations that were forwarded to the Home Office and quickly incorporated into the *Anatomy Act* of 1832, regularising the supply of cadavers.

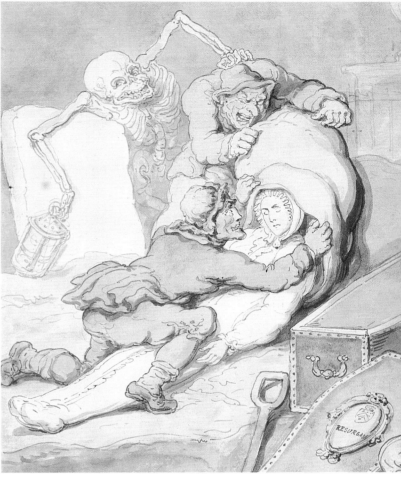

3.14

Contrary to Wakley's accusations, Council was indeed trying to bring about reforms. In 1832 a working party was set up under Sir Astley Cooper of Guy's Hospital (Fig 3.16) to consider the state of the College and the role of its Members. It comprised Sir Anthony Carlisle and George James Guthrie from the Westminster Hospital, Benjamin Travers of St Thomas's, Sir Charles Bell of the Middlesex, and Thomas Copeland and Benjamin Brodie of St Bartholomew's. Their report produced a number of radical proposals, all of which were rejected.

3.15 **Extracts from the diary of a Resurrection Man, 1811–1812**

3.16 Sir Astley Paston Cooper (1768–1841)

The leading surgeon of his day, Cooper was as famous
for his anatomical studies as for his operating and
teaching. Perhaps his most famous work was a treatise
on hernia, published in 1804. His lectures were based
upon sound scientific principles of observation through
dissection and logical deduction of treatment after
a thorough understanding of the physiological,
pathological and surgical principles involved. Students
from around the world attended his lectures. On his
death, the College purchased 1,699 of his anatomical
specimens for £1,500. He is commemorated by a fine
statue in the south transept of St Paul's Cathedral.

By Sir Thomas Lawrence (1769–1830)

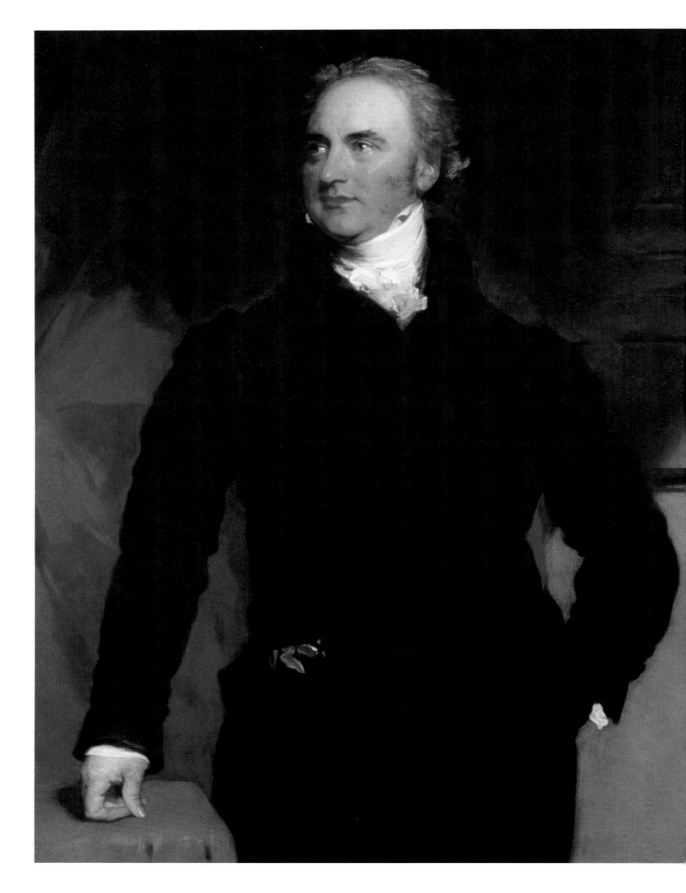

In 1836, upon becoming President for the second time, Astley Cooper convened an extraordinary meeting at which it was agreed that 'No person be recognised as a lecturer on Anatomy and Physiology, Pathology or Surgery in England until he shall have undergone an examination by the Council of the College on two separate days, the first examination on anatomy and physiology, the second on pathology and the principles and practice of surgery'. Nine months later the first candidate came forward: Erasmus Wilson (Fig 3.17).

3.17 Sir William James Erasmus Wilson (1809–1884)

Son of a naval surgeon, Wilson became one of the first 300 Fellows of the Royal College of Surgeons. His friend Thomas Wakley directed his attention to dermatology, the practice of which made Wilson very rich. By shrewd investment, he became even richer. Wilson endowed a Chair in Dermatology in 1869, served as President in 1881, and gave evidence that enabled Wakley to put a stop to flogging in the army. It was Wilson who had Cleopatra's Needle transported to London, and upon his death, he bequeathed £210,000 to the College, a sum that funded the rebuilding works of 1887.

By John Lewis Reilly

3.17

Members of Council wrote down questions, which were put in a glass and shaken up. The candidate drew out one question at a time (Fig 3.18). Having answered all the questions satisfactorily, Wilson passed the examination. The rules were changed for the third candidate, Rutherford Alcock, who was made to give a lecture at short notice on aneurysm. He also passed, but at this stage it was recognised that the process would be too slow to put in place sufficient numbers of teachers.

While a solution was being formulated, the College found itself concerned with serious practical problems. An examination by Sir John Soane, the honorary architect to the College, discovered that Dance's building had serious structural defects: the museum and the lecture theatre were too small, and an almost complete reconstruction was required. Somewhat to the chagrin of

3.18 Cartoon of an examination in the College
By George Cruikshank (1792–1878)

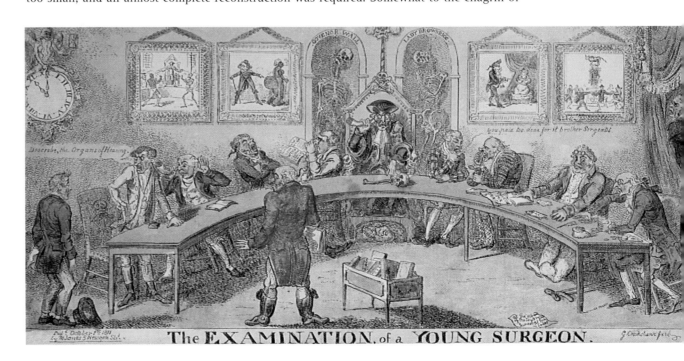

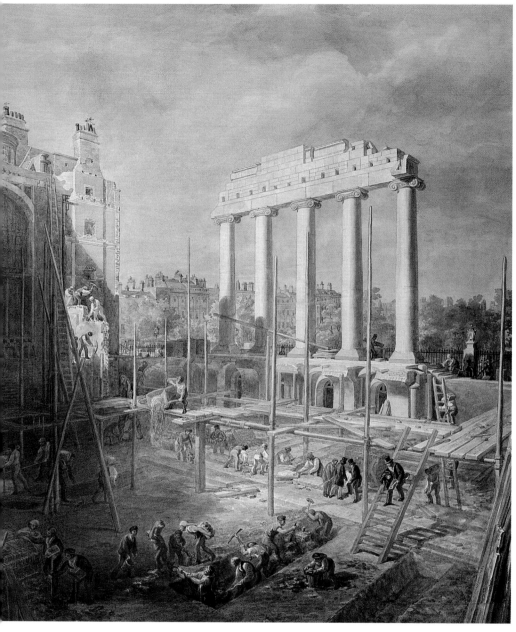

Soane, a public competition was held in 1833 and was won by Charles Barry (Fig 3.19), who designed the Travellers' Club and was later to build the Houses of Parliament. The new building was considerably larger, thanks to the recent purchase of property at 40 Lincoln's Inn Fields. Barry designed a new library, approached by a grand staircase, which is essentially unchanged today (Fig 3.20).

In 1843 the College tried to raise its educational standards through a new Charter (Fig 3.21) that established the Fellowship of the Royal College of Surgeons (FRCS). Initially, 300 Fellows were elected from among the College's existing Members. Thereafter, to gain the FRCS Members had to take a higher examination. Along with this new scheme came an end to life tenure for members of Council; now they would be elected by the Fellows, with the possibility of re-election for a second term. Members of the Court of Examiners also became subject to limited tenure, at the pleasure of Council. At the same time, the name of the College was changed from the Royal College of Surgeons in London to The Royal College of Surgeons of England, reflecting an extension of its ambitions beyond the City of London.

The new Charter did not please Wakley or George James Guthrie (Fig 3.22), Wellington's medical adviser and hero of Waterloo; he wrote to the House of Commons asking to be heard at the Bar of the House. Meanwhile, the principal medical officers of the army and navy sent in a long list of names, demanding that virtually all their serving surgeons be granted the Fellowship.

3.19 Rebuilding the College

View of the demolition of George Dance's building and preparatory work for the new building designed by Sir Charles Barry. Barry retained the portico but realigned the position of the columns to match the new extended façade.

Watercolour by George Scharf, 1834

3.20 Grand staircase and entrance hall of the building by Sir Charles Barry as it was in 1900

Civilian Members of the College who were not nominated were furious. Wakley organised protest meetings and became even more vituperative in the *Lancet*; although some 240 additional Fellows were accepted, the changes went ahead. The examination was simplified. There were still to be two parts – one in basic sciences, one in surgery, pathology and therapeutics – but now each part would have a written paper and an oral examination

3.20

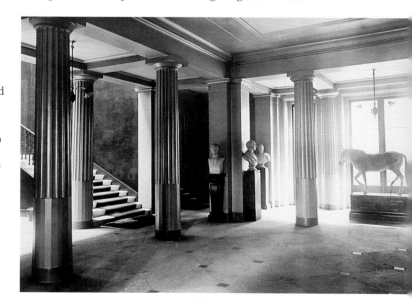

3.21 Charter of 1843

3.22 George James Guthrie (1785–1856)

A member of the College at 16, Guthrie served as
medical officer to a regiment in Canada and in the
Peninsular War, returned in 1814, and was recalled
by Wellington for Waterloo. He was a great military
surgeon and introduced radical changes in the
treatment of gunshot wounds. On his return to London,
he began a course of lectures that was perpetuated
for 20 years for all medical officers of the public
service. He was a pioneer in ophthalmic and prostatic
surgery. Guthrie served on Council from 1824 to 1856
and was President in 1833, 1841 and 1854. This rare
daguerreotype is in the College collection.

By Henry Room

3.23 Sir Richard Owen (1804–1892)

Having been prosector in anatomy to John Abernethy
at St Bartholomew's, Owen became a Member of the
College in 1826 and was appointed assistant conservator
of the museum in 1827 at a salary of £30 per quarter.
He attended Georges Cuvier's lectures in Paris in 1831,
made his reputation with his *Memoir on the Pearly
Nautilus*, was elected a Fellow of the Royal Society in
1834, and appointed Professor of Comparative Anatomy
at St Bartholomew's. More than anyone else, Owen's
scientific researches and series of popular lectures
established the College as a centre for comparative
anatomy. To the museum came gifts of fossils and
specimens from all over the world, including many of
those recovered by Darwin in the explorations of HMS
Beagle. He designed the models of extinct animals for
the Crystal Palace, and moved to the British Museum
(Natural History) in 1856. He helped Livingstone write
his *Missionary Travels* and was involved in an acerbic
dispute with Charles Darwin and Thomas Huxley
concerning natural selection.

By William Etty (1787–1849)

on dissections and operations. Twenty-four
candidates passed the first new examination
in December 1844.

While these negotiations were underway, William
Clift, the loyal disciple of John Hunter, retired.
Clift was succeeded by his son-in-law, Richard
Owen (Fig 3.23), who became the foremost
comparative anatomist of his time and later head
of the Department of Natural History at the British
Museum. As Conservator, he made the Hunterian Museum and the
College famous by his annual lectures and his celebrated dispute with
Charles Darwin over natural selection.

At this stage, the College existed primarily as an examining body of aspiring general practitioner
surgeons with its MRCS, and of teachers with its FRCS. Teaching and training were still
secondary activities. John Hunter's great tradition of research was confined to the work in the
museum of Owen and his successors who – although they were to include over the years such
great names as Sir William Flower, John Quekett, Sir Arthur Keith and Frederic Wood Jones –
were increasingly removed from the world of workaday surgery.

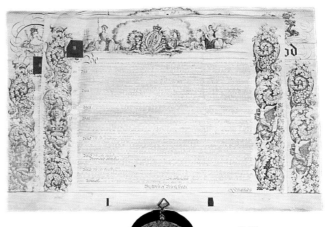

3.21

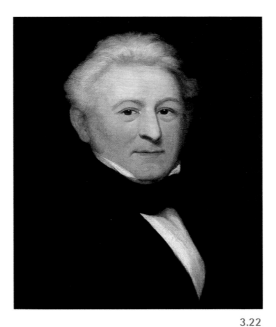

3.22

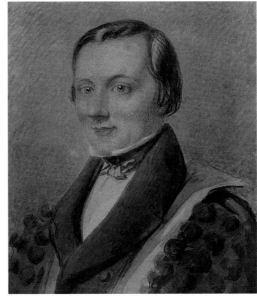

3.23

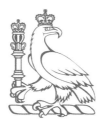

CHAPTER 4

An Era *of* Surgical Evolution

4.1 Sir Thomas Spencer Wells (1818–1897)

Spencer Wells studied at Trinity College Dublin and St Thomas's Hospital. He became a Member of the College in 1841, served in the Royal Naval Hospital in Malta for six years, and was one of a group of naval surgeons to be made a Fellow without examination in 1844. He began in civilian practice as an ophthalmologist but left for the Crimean War in 1855, where he had extensive experience treating abdominal injuries. On his return, he became an expert on ovariotomy. He is credited with the design of the artery forceps that bear his name.

By Rudolph Lehmann

4.2 Spencer Wells artery forceps

This is the true 'Spencer Wells' still in use. In this second version, Spencer Wells moved the ratchet distally and eliminated the gap between the handles to prevent omentum becoming entangled. Thanks to the catch, the forceps could be applied to larger vessels and ligated when convenient, rather than immediately; for smaller vessels the powerful crushing of the jaws sealed them and no ligature was necessary.

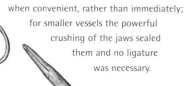

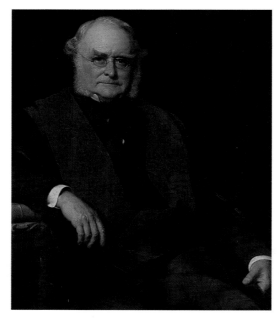

Midway through the 19th century, the practice of surgery was transformed by four discoveries: anaesthesia, accurate dissection and haemostasis, the bacterial origin of infection, and the microscopic study of pathology. The College was closely involved in all of these developments. They quickly led to an increase in the range and scope of surgery and, before long, to the growth of specialisation within surgery.

Anaesthesia was introduced in 1846. Its importance to the practice of medicine and to the history of the College merits more detailed discussion later in this book (Chapter 12).

Because anaesthesia removed the pain from surgery, the operator had more time to dissect carefully and gently, and to stop bleeding by precise ligature avoiding the erroneous inclusion of nerves and other tissues. Arterial forceps, which formerly required bi-manual control, became uni-manual and self-holding owing to the ratchet of Adolphe Charrière; this innovation was introduced in 1858 and adapted over the next 15 years, most notably by Thomas Spencer Wells (Figs 4.1 and 4.2). It was soon evident that crushing by haemostat alone was sufficient to seal small vessels permanently. Importantly, catgut ligatures were rendered sterile and stronger yet absorbable as a result of the dedicated research of Joseph Lister, a keen microscopist (Fig 4.3).

4.3 Lord Lister (1827–1912)

Joseph Lister qualified at University College, passed
the FRCS of England in 1852 and was present in London
when Robert Liston performed his first operation on
a patient anaesthetised with ether. He studied under
James Syme in Edinburgh, took the FRCS Ed in 1855,
and married Syme's eldest daughter. He was elected
to the Regius Chair in Glasgow in 1860, where his
attention was drawn to Louis Pasteur's work, and he
at once began applying antiseptic fluids to surgical
wounds, publishing his results in 1867. He returned
to the Chair of Clinical Surgery in Edinburgh two years
later, and was invited to King's College Hospital in
London in 1877 to modernise its antiseptic techniques.
He was Vice-President in 1886, but declined to be
nominated for the office of President. He was elected
President of the Royal Society in 1895.

By Walter William Ouless

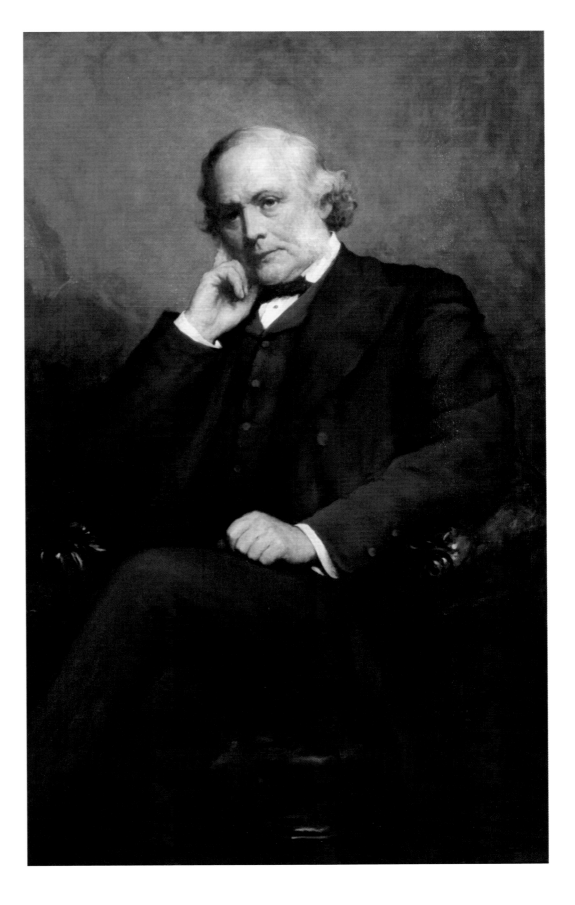

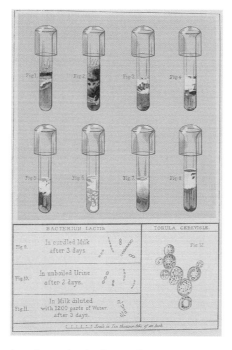

4.4 Lord Lister's drawings of micro-organisms

4.5 The carbolic acid steam spray

In 1865 Lister applied Louis Pasteur's discovery of the souring of wine by micro-organisms to deduce that microbes in the air were the source of wound infections (Fig 4.4). By steeping his hands, instruments and dressings in phenol (carbolic acid) and dispersing it as a spray (Figs 4.5 and 4.6), Lister reduced the infection of fresh wounds drastically. He published the results of his use of antiseptics in 1867, and those who followed his instructions were able to practise safer and more predictable surgery. Some 25 years later, German and French surgeons replaced chemical with thermal sterilisation techniques (known as asepsis), for all but the patient's skin and surgeon's hands, which, for obvious reasons, still required antiseptic preparation.

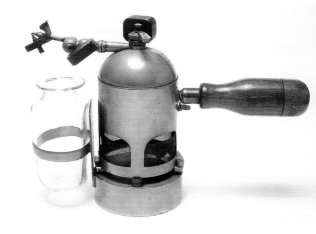

4.5

Although they knew nothing of bacteria, other researchers of the time, such as Oliver Wendell Holmes and Ignaz Semmelweis, discovered that scrupulous cleanliness helped to prevent infection. Thomas Spencer Wells, upon returning from the Crimean War in 1856, devoted himself to improving the results of the operation to remove cysts of the ovary. In addition to meticulous haemostasis, Wells insisted on thorough cleaning and at the end of every operation washed out the abdomen with copious amounts of distilled water.

4.6 The 'donkey-engine' carbolic acid spray, c. 1871

Desiring more spray for major operations, this large apparatus proved satisfactory. Cumbersome to transport (often in Lister's open carriage), it became an object of public ridicule and was given the name of 'donkey-engine'. Lister was glad to replace it with the steam spray.

Technical developments in cutting and staining thin sections of tissue led to a new understanding of the microscopic nature of surgical diseases and to a logical basis for treatment. Among the foremost practitioners in this field were Sir James Paget (Fig 4.7) of St Bartholomew's Hospital and Sir Jonathan Hutchinson (Fig 4.8) of The London Hospital, each in time to become President of the College.

It was through the new microscopic pathology that dentistry became a discrete scientific profession, leading to dentists joining the College. The credit is due to the efforts of a small group of dental

4.7 Sir James Paget (1814–1899)

Even as a medical student, Paget had been interested in microscopy. He had discovered *Trichinella spiralis* in the muscle of a cadaver, although Richard Owen examined the specimen, recognised it as a nematode, and took credit for the discovery. Paget is remembered in the eponymous disease of the bone and nipple. He served as President in 1875.

Cartoon by Spy, Vanity Fair

4.8 Sir Jonathan Hutchinson (1828–1913)

In addition to being a busy general surgeon, Jonathan Hutchinson was a notable ophthalmologist, venereologist, dermatologist and pathologist. He published nine volumes of his own researches in a series of *Archives of Surgery* and founded his own museum as well as the Medical Protection Society. He was President of the College in 1889.

Cartoon by Spy, Vanity Fair

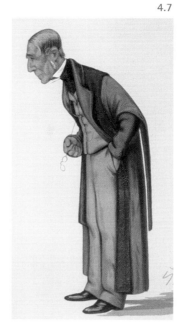
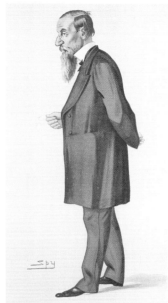
4.7   4.8

surgeons led by John Tomes (see also Fig 13.1) who, having qualified as a doctor and trained as a surgeon, applied himself to the microscopic study of disorders of the teeth and gums. He founded the Odontological Society and eventually overcame much opposition to persuade the College to hold examinations 'for the purpose of testing the fitness of persons to practice as dentists'; this led to the first Licentiates in Dental Surgery in 1860. Today, there are two faculties of dentistry within the College.

The next 20 years saw the new surgery flourish (Fig 4.9). Antiseptic surgery yielded to asepsis. The carbolic spray as an antiseptic was given up in favour of asepsis and scrupulous cleanliness. Instruments, dressings and operative clothing were sterilised by heat. Surgeons changed their blood-stained frock-coats for autoclaved gowns and began to wear masks and rubber gloves. Year by year, the limits of surgery were extended.

4.9 Council of 1884

The group portrait presented by Thomas Spencer Wells to the College in 1884 captures a critical moment in the history of surgery and of the College: Spencer Wells and William Savory were among the last to oppose Lister, and Paget and Hutchinson were two of the pioneers of histopathology.

Left to right: John Whitaker Hulke, Thomas Bryant, William Cadge, Arthur Edward Durham, Henry Power, George Lawson, Edward Lund, Sir Thomas Spencer Wells, Sir James Paget, John Croft, Sir William Scovell Savory (Vice-President), Sir William MacCormac, John Cooper Forster (President), Edward Trimmer (Secretary), Timothy Holmes (Vice-President), Christopher Heath, Matthew Berkeley Hill, Sir John Eric Erichsen, William Allingham, Sir Thomas Smith, Sydney Jones, John Marshall, Lord Lister, John Wood, Sir Frederic Greville Hallett (Assistant Secretary), Sir Jonathan Hutchinson.

By Henry Jamyn Brooks

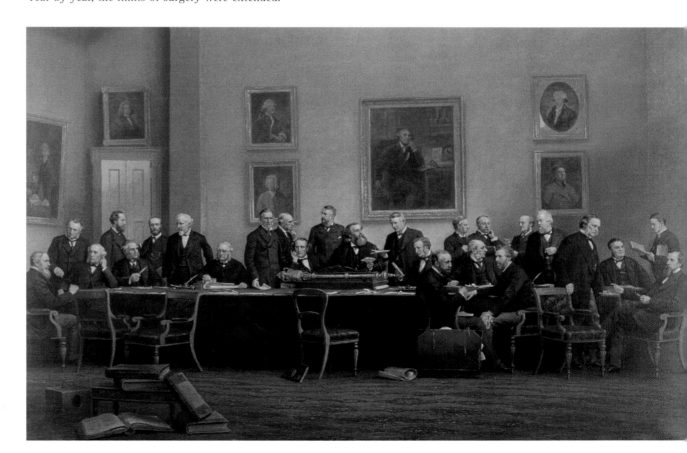

4.10 The Oral Examination

An imaginary scene in the old Council Room during the oral in surgical pathology of the final FRCS examination. The painting was presented to the College in 1948. Left to right: Edward Lund (1823–1898), Sir William MacCormac (1836–1901), first and second candidates, John Wood (1825–1891), third candidate at back, Sir Jonathan Hutchinson (1828–1913), John Marshall (1818–1850), Frederick Le Gros Clark (1811–1892). Lund practised in Manchester and was a keen Listerian. Wood was said to have 'almost lived in the dissecting room' and took up Lister's method towards the end of his career. Marshall had been Liston's assistant and was among the first to recognise that cholera was spread by drinking water. They were a formidable group, but they never performed examinations together.

By Henry Jamyn Brooks, 1894

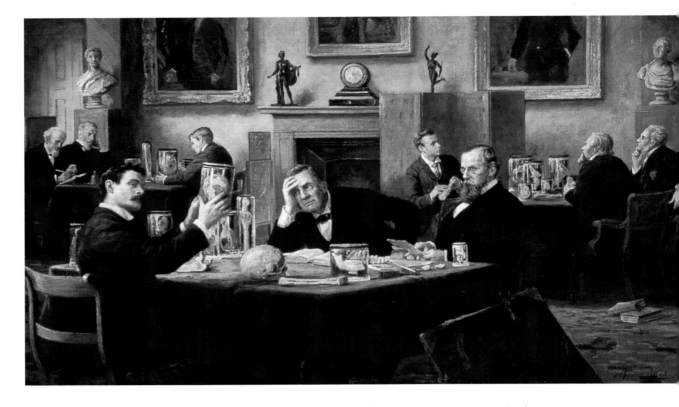

4.11 The Examination Hall on the Thames Embankment

This hall was opened in 1886 for the new conjoint qualification of the Royal Colleges of Physicians and Surgeons. Later it was enlarged to provide laboratories. The building was sold to the Institute of Electrical Engineers in 1908.

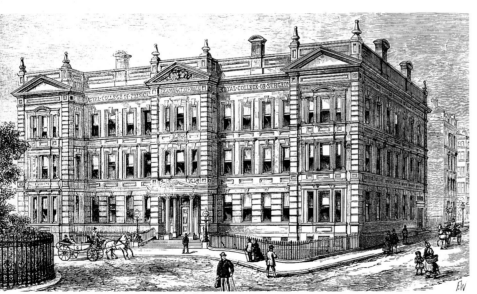

4.12 The Victoria Cross

The Victoria Cross was instituted after the Crimean War in 1856. Among the first to be honoured were two members of this College: James Mouat at the Charge of the Light Brigade, and Thomas Hale at Sebastopol. Since then it has been awarded to 15 other Licentiates, Members and Fellows, one of whom (Arthur Martin-Leake) received it twice.

(Courtesy Royal Army Medical Corps Museum, Aldershot)

The College retained its duty of ensuring through its examinations that surgeons were appropriately trained (Fig 4.10). In those days, teaching was not believed to be its primary business; nevertheless, as early as 1890, in combination with the Royal College of Physicians, joint research laboratories were established in the new Examination Hall on the Thames Embankment (Fig 4.11). Here, some of the most famous names in medicine received their early training in the disciplines of research. It was here also that the fundamental work was undertaken that led to immunisation against typhoid and diphtheria.

The Boer War

In 1899 war broke out in South Africa and stretched the newly formed Royal Army Medical Corps (RAMC) to the limits of its resources. As more surgeons were needed in the Cape, many civilian surgeons volunteered. From Council went Frederick Treves, Watson Cheyne, Jonathan Hutchinson, Victor Horsley, Anthony Bowlby, George Makins and Sir William MacCormac. With them went a large number of medical students for whom it had been decreed that time spent as an assistant attached to the army in South Africa would count for the equivalent period of medical or surgical hospital practice. Many surgeons, however, succumbed to typhoid and never returned; the new antisera were effective, but in short supply.

4.12

For the first time in a major military campaign, the principles of the new surgery – anaesthesia, antisepsis and haemostasis – were put to a stringent test.

4.13 Arthur Martin-Leake (1874–1953)

Trained at University College Memorial Hospital, Martin-Leake left his hospital position to serve under Baden-Powell as Surgeon-Captain, and won his first Victoria Cross for going 'out into the firing line to dress a wounded man under very heavy fire from about forty Boers only 100 yards off. When he had done all he could for him, he went over to a badly wounded officer, and while trying to place him in a more comfortable position, he was shot about three times'. He studied for the FRCS while convalescing, passed in 1903, and won his second Victoria Cross at the First Battle of Ypres for 'rescuing, while exposed to constant fire, a large number of the wounded who were lying close to the enemy's trenches'.

(Courtesy Royal Army Medical Corps Museum, Aldershot)

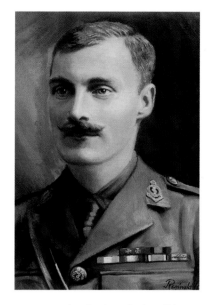

4.14 Sir Frederick Treves (1853–1923)

School friend of Thomas Hardy, Treves was a popular teacher and anatomist who carried out important studies on the peritoneum just when laparotomy was becoming safe. He will always be remembered for his kindness to the 'Elephant Man', Joseph Merrick. Treves, who had been one of the first to abandon the carbolic spray, led a field hospital that treated casualties from the Battle of Colenso and the subsequent relief of Ladysmith, services for which he was knighted.

Cartoon by Spy, Vanity Fair

4.15 Sir Rickman John Godlee (1849–1925)

Godlee studied under his uncle Joseph Lister in Edinburgh, was the first to discover the *Streptococcus* in pus from an abscess, wrote and illustrated a magnificent *Atlas of Human Anatomy* based on his own dissections, and was the first to remove a glioma of the brain. He was President in 1912 and gave an inaugural address to the American College of Surgeons.

By Alan Bacon, 1923

They proved remarkably successful. Using a combination of antiseptic solutions, mainly carbolic and hydrogen peroxide, the surgical teams reduced the mortality from gunshot wounds even when the great cavities – the head, thorax and abdomen – were involved. There were other technical innovations: rail transport was used to evacuate the wounded speedily and smoothly, and intravenous saline and X-rays were introduced for the first time. The medical officers in the new RAMC were respected as professionals and quickly showed that, even though they were technically non-combatants, they were far from wanting in courage. No fewer than nine Victoria Crosses (Fig 4.12) for valour were won by doctors during this campaign, including Arthur Martin-Leake who was the first to be awarded the Victoria Cross on two occasions (Fig 4.13).

If the Boer War vindicated the new surgery, the ultimate seal of approval came just after the war when London was packed with visitors for the coronation of Edward VII. Two days before he was due to be crowned, the King fell critically ill. An appendix abscess, brewing for weeks, was on the point of rupture. Sir Frederick Treves (Fig 4.14) was sent for and in consultation with Lord Lister and Sir Thomas Smith agreed that an operation was absolutely necessary. The King protested that he could not let his people down, he must go to Westminster Abbey. 'In that case, Sir,' said Treves, 'it will be as a corpse.'

The King was overweight, chesty and an inveterate smoker. His abscess was deeply seated. Even today the operation would be dangerous. Treves managed with some difficulty to persuade the Queen to leave the room, took off his coat,

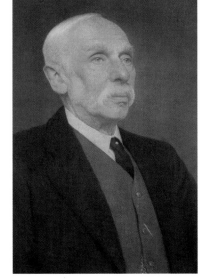

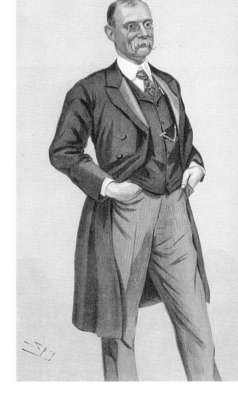

scrubbed up and drained the abscess. The King recovered. Never had the value of the new surgery been demonstrated so dramatically, and Treves became famous overnight. The College shared in his glory. Surgery came to be seen as yet another example of the marvels of science, along with engineering and electricity.

4.14

The first decade of the 20th century was a golden time for surgery and the College. As the College celebrated its first centenary honorary fellowships were introduced and awarded primarily to distinguished surgeons from overseas. In 1913 Sir Rickman Godlee (Fig 4.15) was host to a notable

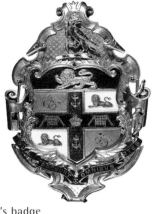

4.16 The President's badge

This was presented by Sir John Tweedy (1849–1924) who became a popular President, cemented the friendship with the Worshipful Company of Barbers, and instituted the Thomas Vicary Lectures.

4.17 Sir Anthony Bowlby (1855–1929)

Sir Anthony Bowlby is probably best remembered for his efforts during the First World War, when he rose to Director-General of the Army Medical Service, and finally to adviser on surgery for the whole of the British area. His greatest contribution was his insistence that surgery be undertaken at the front, changing casualty clearing stations into large hospitals. He was elected President of the College in 1920.

By Dorofield Hardy, 1930
(copy of original by W Llewellyn)

4.18 Sir George Makins (1853–1933)

Makins served in both the Boer War and the First World War, where he was adviser on surgery to the forces and established a research centre at which new methods of wound treatment were examined. He left France in 1917 and was appointed chairman of a commission to report on British station hospitals in India, a responsibility that entailed travelling all over that country. He served as President of the College from 1917 to 1920.

By Mary Pownall
Bromet, 1930

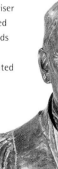

collection of visitors who were made Honorary Fellows and, in the same year, Godlee went to the United States to address the inauguration of the American College of Surgeons. In 1904, Sir John Tweedy presented to the College an enamelled gold badge to be worn by the President (Fig 4.16).

In 1902 Sir Henry Morris announced that he had made a gift to both the College and the Royal College of Physicians in the amount of £100,000 to be used for research into cancer. A joint Cancer Research Committee was set up to establish what became the Imperial Cancer Research Fund. A handsome endowment for educational scholarships was received from Eliza Macloghlin.

The First World War

At the outbreak of the First World War, many Fellows joined the new Territorial Medical Service and were sent to France. They included Sir Anthony Bowlby (Fig 4.17), Sir George Makins (Fig 4.18) and Sir Berkeley Moynihan, all of whom later became Presidents of the College.

To their consternation, the older surgeons found that the methods that had been so successful in South Africa did not seem to work in France. The wounds caused by heavy machine guns and artillery were more severe than the 'clean' Mauser bullet wounds seen in the veldt. Worse, the mud of Flanders brought a new hazard caused by the spores of *Clostridium welchii*, which were present in manure and resistant to most antiseptics. Gas gangrene now appeared on an alarming scale. It took some weeks before the correct treatment was identified as wide excision of all dead and devitalised tissue so that there would be nowhere for the spores to reside.

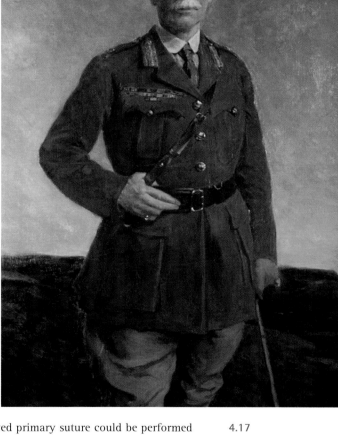

4.17

The wound was then left unclosed, and delayed primary suture could be performed five or six days later. Bowlby and Makins insisted that, contrary to official policy, this life-saving wound excision should be performed as soon after the injury as possible. Evacuating the wounded soldier back to base hospital, even by train, took so long that fatal infection was almost inevitable.

Another unexpected lesson was the management of abdominal wounds. Conservative treatment had sometimes been successful in South Africa, but proved lethal in

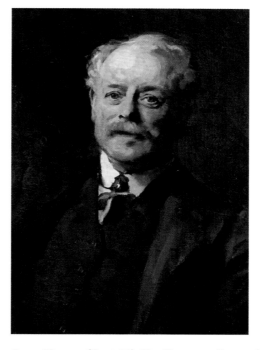

4.19 Sir Robert Jones (1858–1933)

Even before he had qualified at Liverpool, Jones was used to assisting his maternal uncle Hugh Owen Thomas. He was appointed to the Royal Southern Hospital in 1889 and provided casualty service for the 10,000 workmen engaged in digging the Manchester Ship Canal. He was responsible for the army's orthopaedic services during the First World War.

By Frank Copnall

Flanders. All penetrating wounds demanded a laparotomy; again, the earlier this operation could be undertaken, the better the outcome. The consequence of these findings was a need for more surgeons to operate in the field hospitals as well as back at base. Along with the changes in the management of gunshot injuries, there came a wide, if grudging, acknowledgement that specialists and specialist teams could achieve better results than generalists.

The most significant of these specialist developments was a splint introduced by Robert Jones (Fig 4.19) that was invented by his uncle, Hugh Owen Thomas (Fig 4.20). The Thomas splint could be applied to fractures of the femur by medical orderlies at the regimental aid post in the trenches. It lessened the damage from the jolting that was inevitable in evacuating the wounded soldier. Routine use of the Thomas splint reduced mortality from fractures of the femur from 60 to 30 per cent. Jones later published his own unofficial handbook on the correct management of wounds involving joints. The handbook proved to be so popular with front-line surgeons that it attracted the notice of the War Office, which set Jones up in a 500-bedded military orthopaedic hospital in Liverpool. Specialisation, at least in orthopaedics, now had the stamp of approval.

4.20 Hugh Owen Thomas (1834–1891)

The last of a long line of Welshmen who combined farming with bone-setting, he was the first of his family to obtain a medical qualification in 1857 and had a large practice in the poorest district of Liverpool where he exercised his knowledge of orthopaedics in free Sunday clinics.

By H Fleury

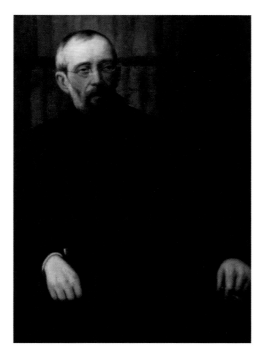

The seeds of other great surgical specialities were also sown in the military hospitals of the First World War. British thoracic surgery effectively started when George Gask (see also Fig 15.21) found that he could safely open the chest for gunshot injuries; nevertheless, without antibiotics empyema was an all too common sequel.

Plastic surgery, particularly the management of burns and the repair of injuries to the face and jaw, emerged as a specialty of its own. Sir Harold Gillies (see also Fig 15.17), a New Zealander working with a team of surgeons from all over the British Empire, developed methods of replacing lost tissue with full-thickness flaps of ingenious design. To record the stages of facial reconstruction, Gillies enlisted Henry Tonks, a surgeon-turned-artist, who made pastel drawings of the patients (Fig 4.21).

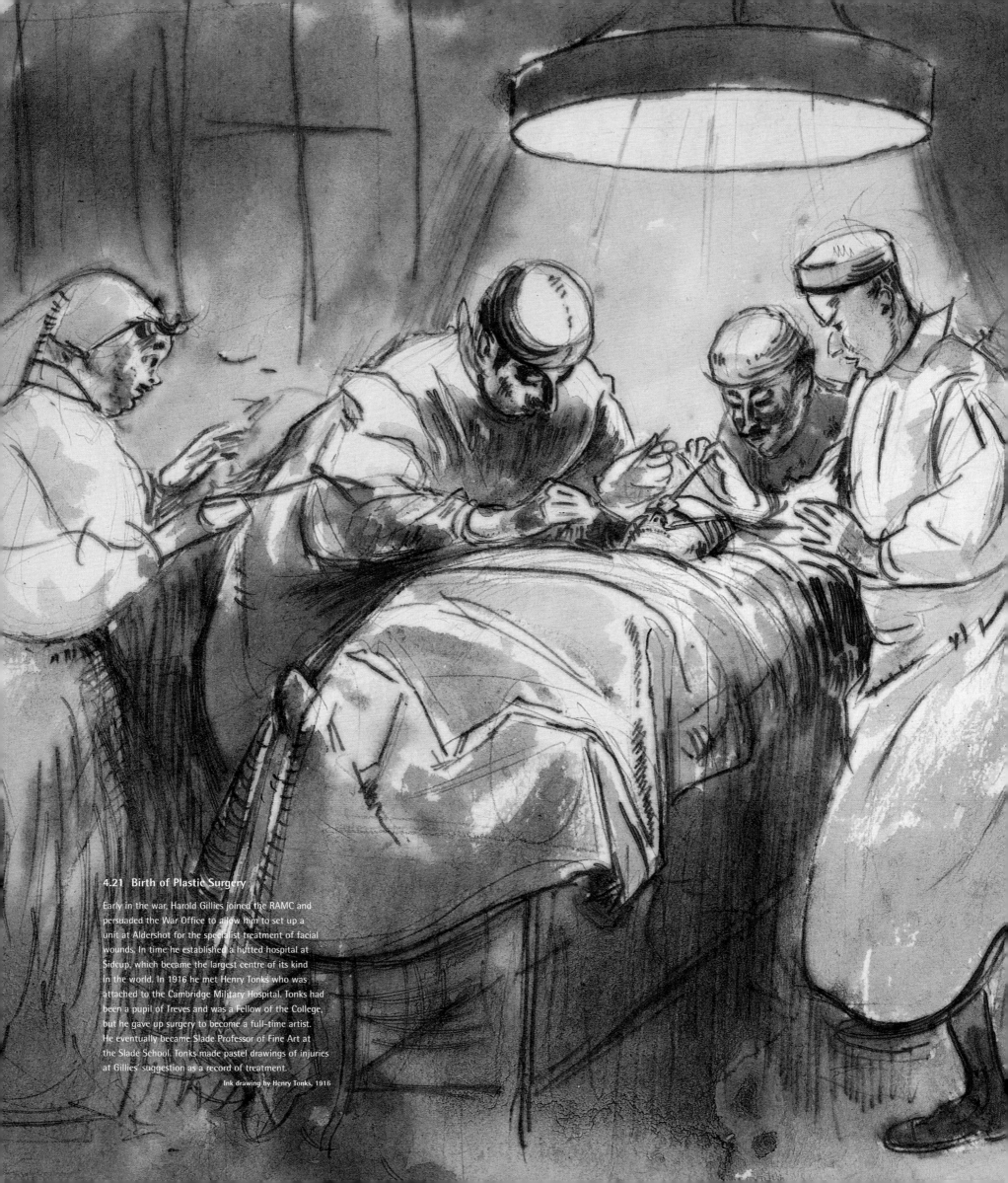

4.21 Birth of Plastic Surgery

Early in the war, Harold Gillies joined the RAMC and persuaded the War Office to allow him to set up a unit at Aldershot for the specialist treatment of facial wounds. In time he established a hutted hospital at Sidcup, which became the largest centre of its kind in the world. In 1916 he met Henry Tonks who was attached to the Cambridge Military Hospital. Tonks had been a pupil of Treves and was a Fellow of the College, but he gave up surgery to become a full-time artist. He eventually became Slade Professor of Fine Art at the Slade School. Tonks made pastel drawings of injuries at Gillies' suggestion as a record of treatment.

Ink drawing by Henry Tonks, 1916

4.22 Lord Moynihan (1865–1936)

Having trained in Leeds, Berkeley Moynihan went on to become consulting surgeon there as well as Professor of Clinical Surgery. He served on the Board of Examiners and on the Council, the latter from 1912 to 1933. He was elected President for six years in succession, 1926–31, and held the office of chairman of the editorial committee of the *British Journal of Surgery* from its inception in 1913 until his death.

By Richard Jack, 1928

4.23 Sir George Buckston Browne (1850–1945)

Buckston Browne had been private assistant to Sir Henry Thompson, the famous lithotomist. He never took the FRCS, but instead earned a great reputation (and a considerable fortune) from treating urethral strictures and stones in the bladder, which in those days were very common. Thompson enjoyed a distinguished social life, and through him Buckston Browne learned to appreciate the arts and fine dining. Upon his retirement, and after having lost his son in the First World War, he devoted himself to public benefactions. In 1928 he bought Charles Darwin's house at Downe and presented it to the British Association as a national memorial. In response to a request from Sir Arthur Keith, he bought 13 acres adjoining the Darwin estate, built the Buckston Browne Farm, and presented it to the College.

By Charles L Hartnell

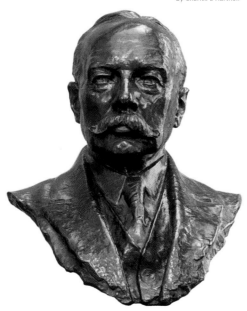

After the War

In 1919 the College was consulted concerning the establishment of the Ministry of Health, and President Sir George Makins was appointed to serve on the consultative committee.

After a distinguished service in the war, Lord Moynihan (Fig 4.22) became President in 1926. He was the first Fellow to be elected President who worked and lived outside the sphere of the London teaching hospitals, thus making an inroad for regional surgeons in the governance of the College. He founded the Association of Surgeons of Great Britain and Ireland and the *British Journal of Surgery*. He was a great ambassador for British surgery internationally as well, travelling to the United States to present a mace to the American College inscribed 'from the consulting surgeons of the British Armies to the American College of Surgeons in memory of mutual work and good fellowship in the European War 1914–18'. His extensive travels convinced him of the value of surgical research, then prominent in Germany and the United States, and he was determined to bring the College to the forefront in this field. The College began to build surgical laboratories and establish research scholarships. The starting point was a series of generous donations from George Buckston Browne (Fig 4.23).

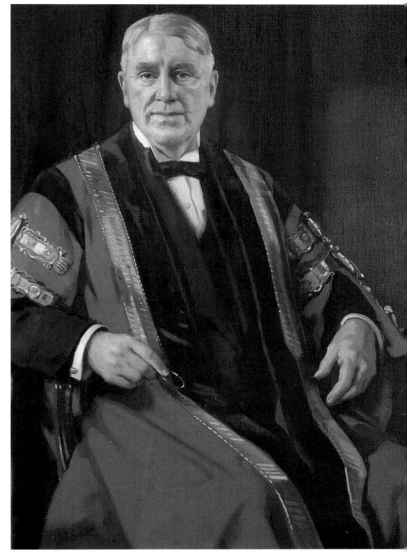

4.22

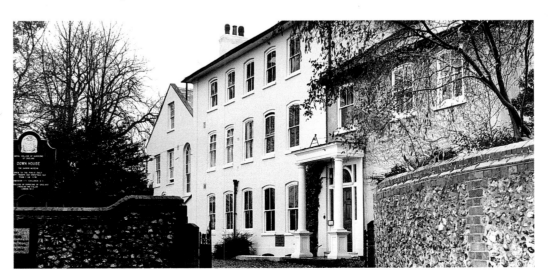

4.24 **Down House**

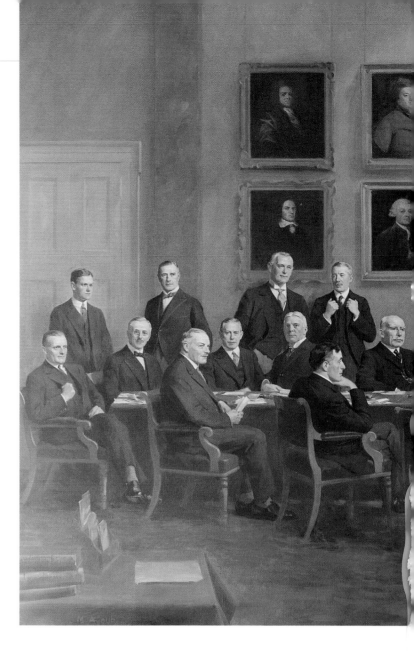

4.25 Sir Arthur Keith (1866–1955)

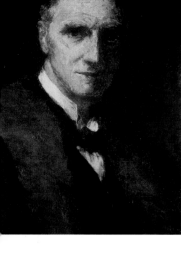

Keith was Conservator of the Hunterian Museum from 1908 to 1933, during which time he helped revive the scientific activities of the College through his lectures and popular writings on anatomy and anthropology. His journalism won him much public renown. Keith was appointed the first Master of the Buckston Browne Farm in 1933 and supervised its research until his death in 1955.

By Walter William Ouless, 1928

Buckston Browne was a great admirer of Charles Darwin. In 1928, he purchased Darwin's old home, Down House (Fig 4.24), and presented it to the British Association for the Advancement of Science. It was formally opened in 1929 by Sir Arthur Keith, Conservator of the Hunterian Museum (Fig 4.25). Over the next few months, Buckston Browne was persuaded by Moynihan and Keith to endow a research institute for the College adjacent to Down House. The Buckston Browne Farm occupied two fields, traditionally known as Great and Little Pucklands (from which Rudyard Kipling derived his Puck of Pook's Hill). Further gifts for research were added: Lord Leverhulme began his annual gifts of £1,000; The Prophit Trust gave £10,000; and Sir Louis Baron added £25,000 in 1936.

This period is captured in the group portrait of Council in 1926–27 (Fig 4.26).

Exporting the Examinations

4.27 Sir Frederic Greville Hallett (1860–1933)

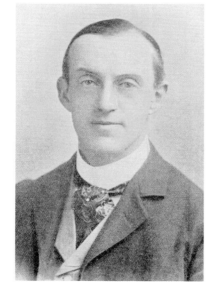

Hallett entered the administration of the College in 1877, was Secretary to the Examination Board of the Conjoint Examination in 1887, and the first Secretary of the Imperial Cancer Research Fund. He was knighted in 1928.

The Hallett Prize was founded in 1935 in his memory and is awarded to the best candidate in the primary Fellowship examination, and subsequently to the top mark in the MRCS.

In addition to this new activity in research the College continued to expand its work as an examining body, which was its only means of maintaining standards. The primary and final Fellowship examinations were held in great respect all over the world. One of the key College people who administered these examinations, and later played a major part in running the research activities of the College, was Sir Frederic Greville Hallett (Fig 4.27) after whom a prize was named for the best candidate in the primary Fellowship.

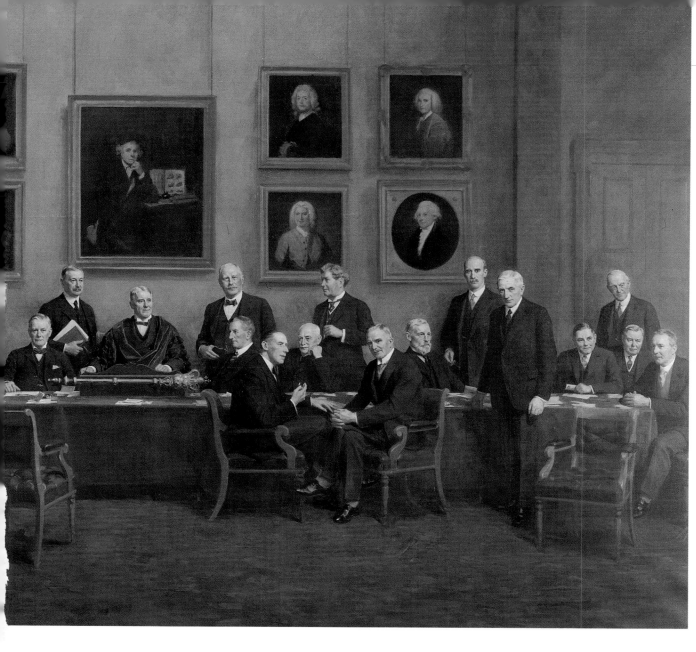

4.26 Council of 1926–27

Left to right: Sir Percy Sargent, Kennedy Cassels (Assistant Secretary), William Thelwall Thomas, John Herbert Fisher, William McAdam Eccles, Robert Pugh Rowlands, Sir Charles Gordon-Watson, Sir Holburt Jacob Waring, George Grey Turner, William Sampson Handley, Sir Anthony Bowlby, Sir Cuthbert Wallace (Vice-President), Sibert Forrest Cowell (Secretary), Lord Moynihan (President), Ernest William Hey Groves, Frances James Steward (Vice-President), Victor Bonney, Sir D'Arcy Power, Sir John Lynn-Thomas, Arthur Henry Burgess, Sir James Berry, Sir Hugh Lett, Wilfred Trotter, Charles Herbert Fagge, Sir Frederic Greville Hallett, Vincent Warren Low, George Ernest Gask.

By Moussa Ayoub, 1927–29

In 1927 a team was invited to Toronto to conduct the first overseas primary FRCS examination. Only nine of the first 23 candidates passed. The following year, the newly inaugurated Australasian College of Surgeons requested that a primary FRCS examination be held in Melbourne; at the first of these, in 1931, ten of the first 20 candidates passed. The examiners returned via Toronto and held another examination there. In due course, arrangements were made to hold the examination in India.

In 1935 President Sir Holburt Waring went to Australia for the formal opening of a new building for the Royal Australasian College of Surgeons, which subsequently set up its own fellowship examinations. However, for many years before and after the Second World War, many Australian and New Zealand surgeons continued to come to the United Kingdom to complete their surgical training and sit the Fellowship examination.

It was at this time that the question was first asked as to whether examinations alone were enough to ensure standards in surgical training. In 1935 Waring asked members of Council to visit and report on hospitals that were seeking approval for surgical training. This was the beginning of the recognition of training posts, which was in time to become formalised by the Hospital Recognition Committee and the Specialist Advisory Committees.

CHAPTER 5

The Second World War

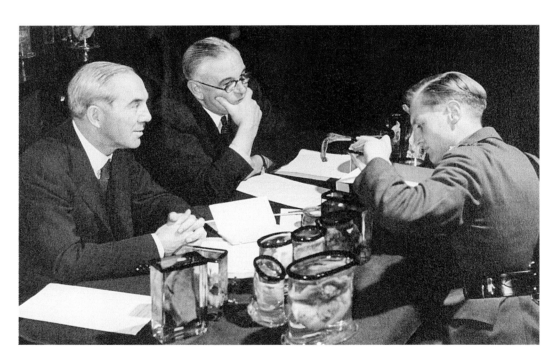

5.1 War-time FRCS examination

Three years before the outbreak of the Second World War, the director general of the Royal Army Medical Corps came to the College to explain to Council the emergency measures that were proposed in the event of another war. Many of those present shared the belief, based on the recent experience of the Spanish Civil War, that the principal hazard of any new conflict would be aerial bombardment. Indiscriminate air raids would result in appalling injuries not only to the armed forces, but also to civilians. A committee of reference was set up to determine how to distribute available surgeons to deal with military and civilian casualties. Temporary hospitals were set up around the major population centres, and each large teaching hospital was made responsible for its own 'sector'.

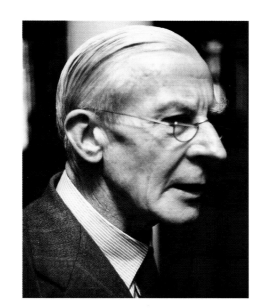

5.2 Lord Adrian (1889–1977)

Edgar Douglas Adrian studied physiology at Cambridge University and later began research on nerves with Keith Lucas. They discovered the 'all-or-none' law in nerve conduction. For this work Adrian was elected to a fellowship at Trinity College in 1913. He received a medical degree in 1915, worked at clinical neurology until 1919 and then returned to Cambridge. His study of the capacity of sense organs to receive different degrees of stimulation culminated in his receipt of the Nobel Prize for Medicine jointly with Sir Charles Scott Sherrington in 1932.

(Courtesy Wellcome Institute Library, London)

One contribution from the College was to have significance that long outlasted the war. Professor John Beattie, head of the College research laboratories, was seconded to Bristol to set up an army blood transfusion service. Eventually, this service developed into the civilian National Blood Transfusion Service, a facility that took surgery another major step forward.

As war drew nearer, the process of getting medical students through their qualifying conjoint examinations was accelerated, and candidates for the Final FRCS were allowed to sit the examination after 12 instead of 27 months' clinical surgical experience (Fig 5.1). The College began to offer teaching courses, initially focused on the basic sciences and designed to help candidates studying for the primary FRCS. The first group of teachers included the neurophysiological genius Edgar Douglas Adrian, later Lord Adrian (Fig 5.2).

On the domestic front, in anticipation of aerial bombing, the College took great care to protect its heritage. More than 7,000 specimens were moved from the Hunterian Collection to what was believed to be the safety of the sub-basement. The library moved 50,000 books to the safety of Aldred Court in Worcestershire. Portraits and other treasures were moved to the Welsh National Library at Aberystwyth. The statue of John Hunter in the hall was bricked up under a concrete roof (Fig 5.3). During the first savage blitz of 1940, the College suffered only minor damage. Then, on the night of 10/11 May 1941, three high explosive bombs fell directly on the College (Fig 5.4 overleaf). The tremendous destruction extended even to the sub-basement, where two-thirds of the Hunterian specimens stored there were destroyed.

5.3 Her Majesty Queen Mary and Lord Webb-Johnson looking at the bricked-up Hunter statue

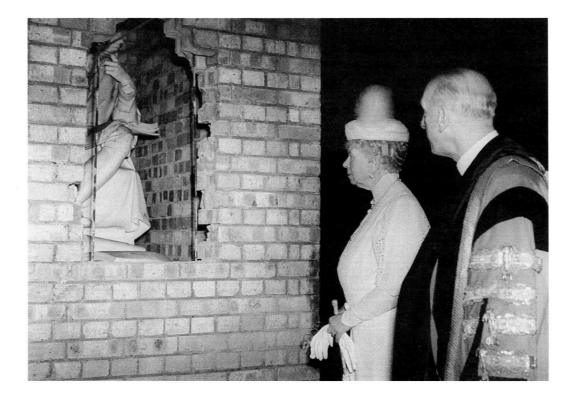

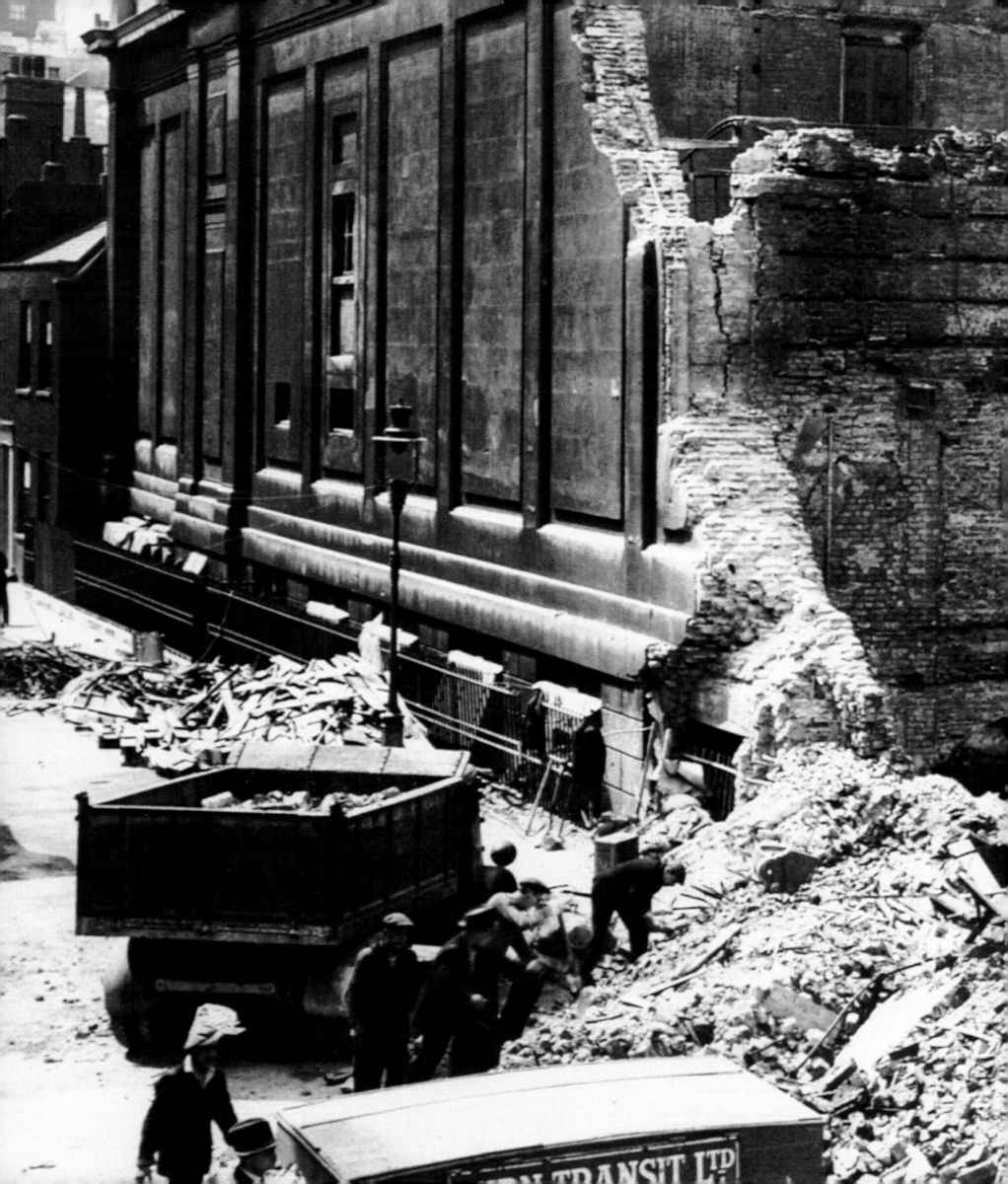

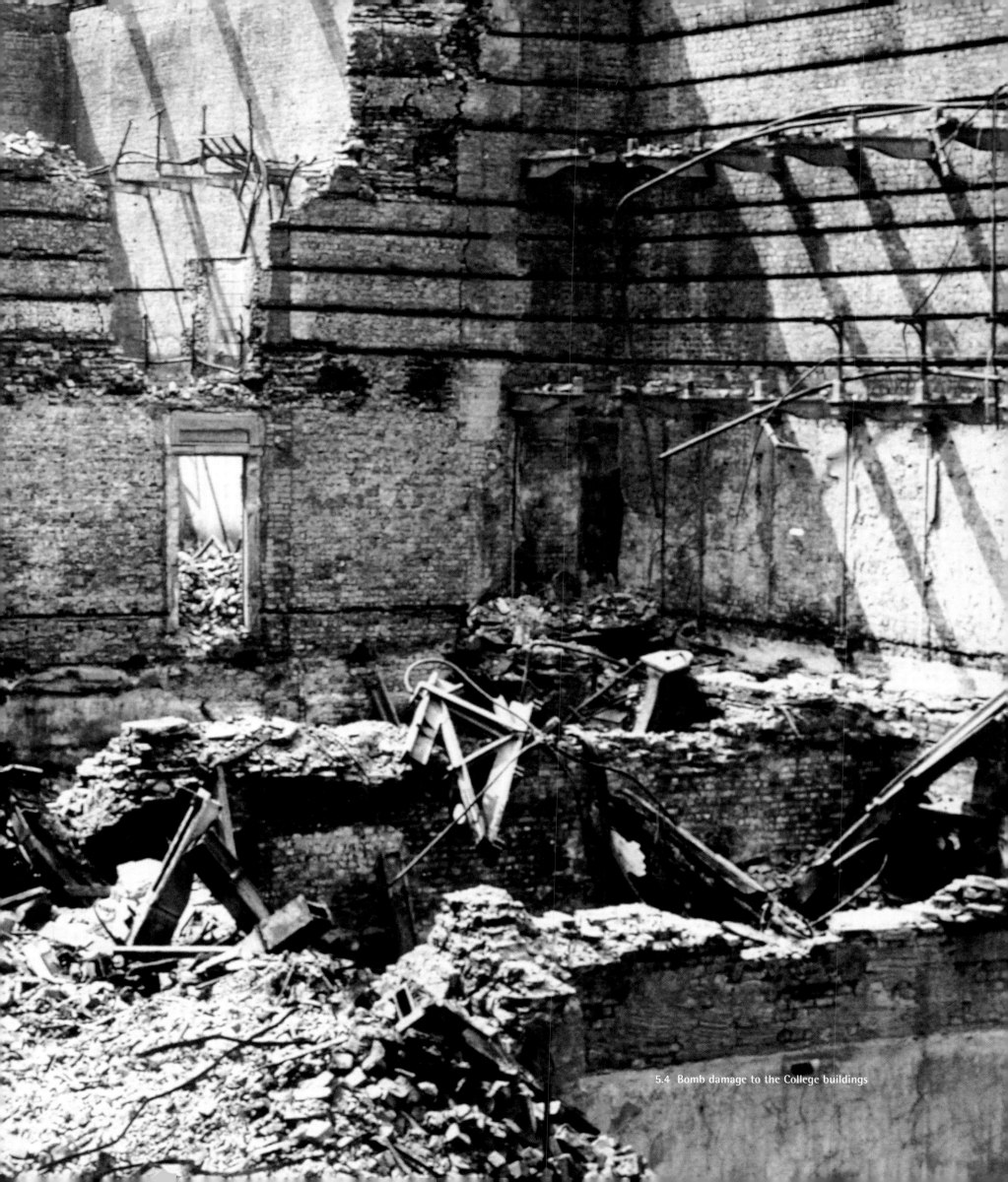

5.4 Bomb damage to the College buildings

5.5 Sir Hugh Lett (1876–1964)

Hugh Lett served as President of the College from 1938 to 1941. He took a personal initiative in the preservation of the College's treasures, and it was he who in 1939 travelled to Aberystwyth to arrange the removal of the most valuable paintings and books to the National Library of Wales. In 1940, he secured a grant from the Rockefeller Foundation to evacuate the library. He married the only daughter of Sir Buckston Browne and took an active interest in his father-in-law's foundations at Downe. After the war, he was elected President of the British Medical Association and worked on the establishment of the National Health Service.

By James Gunn

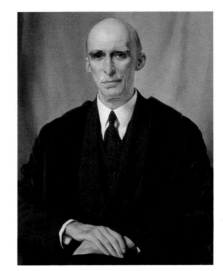

5.5

Fortunately, some 26,000 specimens were saved, but the College was an uninhabitable shell. Sir Hugh Lett, then President (Fig 5.5), was galvanised into action. The surviving specimens were sent to the country in 70 vehicles supplied by the American Ambulance Corps.

Already celebrated for his success in raising funds for the rebuilding of the Middlesex Hospital, Lett's successor as President, Alfred Webb-Johnson (Fig 5.6) threw his energies into four priorities: rebuilding, research, education, and keeping the newly emerging specialties within the body of the College. Webb-Johnson's imaginative vision and his contribution to the survival of the College and its successful post-war development cannot be over-emphasised.

Even with bombs still falling, plans were drawn up for rebuilding the College. Webb-Johnson envisaged making Lincoln's Inn Fields a centre for the medical sciences (Fig 5.7). He tried to persuade the Royal Colleges of Physicians and of Gynaecology and Obstetrics to join The Royal College of Surgeons in creating one multi-disciplinary campus. It was a far-sighted plan but, sadly, came to nothing.

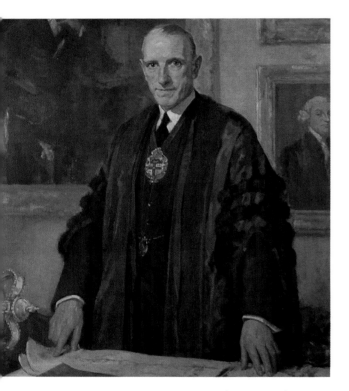

5.6 Lord Webb-Johnson (1880–1958)

Originally from Manchester, Alfred Webb-Johnson came to London in 1907 as resident medical officer at the Middlesex Hospital. He became a consulting surgeon there but was more involved in the administration of the hospital, acting as dean of the medical school for six years and chairman of the re-building committee for ten years.

Webb-Johnson was elected President in 1941 and re-elected seven times. He threw his extraordinary energy firstly into rebuilding the College and secondly into extending its activities. His term of office saw the rebuilding of the College, the introduction of improved ceremonial and monthly dinners to increase interest among Fellows and Members, the introduction of regular programmes of teaching and research, the formation of the special faculties and the endowment of special professorships.

By Francis Hodge

5.7 Floor plans for the proposed Royal Medical Colleges

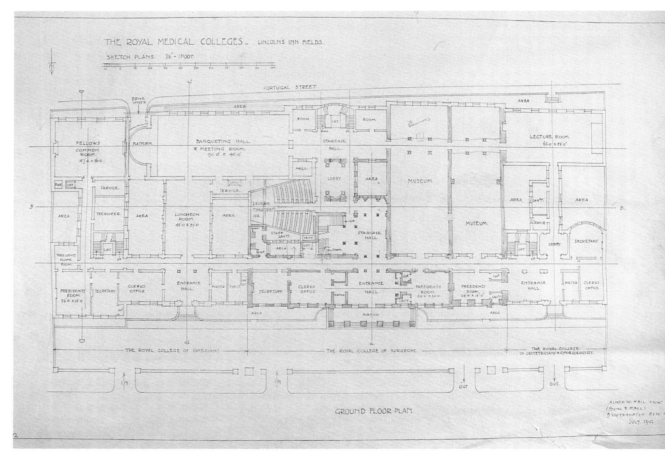

5.7

A new department for ophthalmic research was opened in 1942, and over the next two years professorial chairs were endowed by Sir William Collins in pathology and anatomy. In true Hunterian tradition, these chairs were to incorporate both human and comparative studies. Their first occupants, Rupert Willis and Frederic Wood Jones (Fig 5.8), became famous in their respective fields, and their departments known throughout the world.

Despite the destruction of so much of the fabric of the College, the basic science and surgery courses were expanded and in great demand (Fig 5.9). The College, like the shops of London with their shattered windows and sandbags, continued to offer 'normal service'.

Meanwhile, out in the sector hospitals where the surgical firms from the major teaching hospitals were waiting for civilian casualties, a quiet revolution was taking place in surgical teaching. Routine work continued, and many of these sector hospitals developed into important specialist units, providing specialist training for a new generation of young surgeons. With their chiefs no longer dashing to and from Harley Street, there was time to talk and to teach. A new concept crept in, at first almost unnoticed, that surgical skills could be taught practically, not merely by holding a retractor.

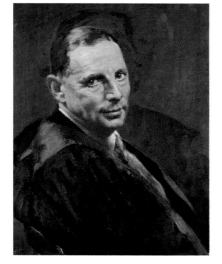

5.8 Professor Frederic Wood Jones (1879–1954)

Frederic Wood Jones was appointed to the Sir William Collins Chair of Comparative and Human Anatomy and as Conservator of the Hunterian Museum, with the aim of restoring the damaged museum. He retired from the Professorship in 1951 but continued as Honorary Conservator until his death in 1954. He qualified as a surgeon after training at the London Hospital in 1904, but had a varied career thereafter, primarily focused on anatomy and natural history.

5.9 Anatomy demonstration conducted at the College during the war

The idea of hands-on skills training rather than observation was not, of course, confined to surgery. Urgent need had forced the Royal Air Force (RAF) to devise a system for turning an 18-year-old schoolboy into a Spitfire pilot in six weeks. People began to ask whether planned, structured courses could do the same for surgery.

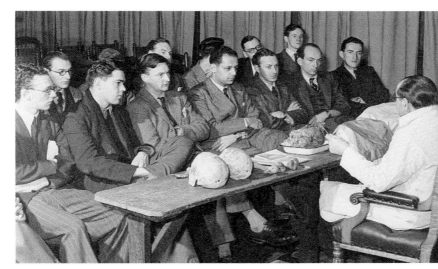

5.9

Webb-Johnson wanted to keep emerging specialties within the body of the College. Some of those that sprang up during the First World War underwent another more vigorous growth spurt during the Second World War, when even more specialties made their first appearance.

In the field of plastic surgery, the work of Archibald McIndoe (see also Fig 15.19) and Sir William Kelsey Fry (see also Fig 13.7) at East Grinstead (Fig 5.10) received widespread publicity and brought the College into close contact with the Blond family of Marks and Spencer's retail fame. Everyone had seen pictures of, or at least had heard about, the remarkable reconstruction of the burnt faces of the heroic young Battle of Britain pilots. It was quickly learned that the sooner an injury or a burn that involved skin loss was seen by an expert,

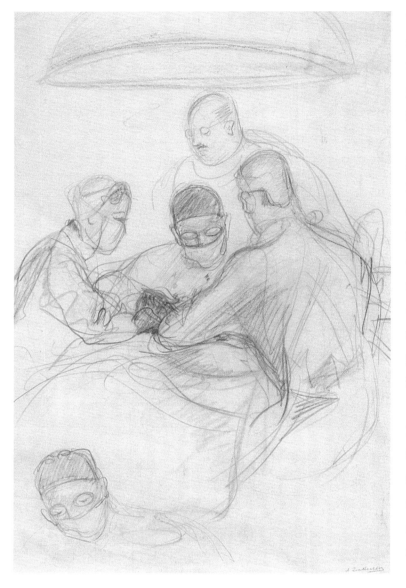

the better the result. Mobile plastic surgery units were established, from which emerged teams that continued to work together long after the war. Equally important was the growing understanding of the pathophysiology of the burned victim and the need for massive fluid replacement.

In neurosurgery, there were equally dramatic advances, led largely by Hugh Cairns from Oxford (Fig 5.11). Again, towards the end of the war, the realisation that better results were obtained by early expert treatment led Cairns to set up neurosurgical units in forward areas. Prevention of head injuries was no less important, and one of Cairns' more rewarding contributions was to insist that military dispatch riders were equipped with crash helmets. Sir Hugh Seddon was developing a new understanding of injuries involving the peripheral nerves: his findings provided a logical basis for appropriate treatment. The rapid advance in anaesthesia was also a major feature of the Second World War.

The lessons of the First World War led to specialist orthopaedic centres for each of the armed forces. In the RAF Sir Reginald Watson-Jones (see also Fig 6.12), Sir Henry Osmond-Clarke (see also Fig 15.6) and others demonstrated that prompt and expert treatment, followed by vigorous rehabilitation, could return young pilots to their cockpits within weeks rather than months.

5.10 Archibald McIndoe operating at Queen Victoria Hospital, East Grinstead

Drawing by Anna Zinkeisen

5.11 Sir Hugh Cairns (1896–1952)

Cairns began his career with an interest in genito-urinary surgery, but turned to neurosurgery working at The London Hospital. In 1937 he established a school of neurosurgery at Oxford and devoted himself to teaching and research; his advice greatly influenced Lord Nuffield's benefactions to the Oxford medical school. During the war, he devised a crash helmet and leg shield for motorcyclists that saved many dispatch riders from injury. He also planned mobile operating theatres for neurosurgery that were invaluable in the fast-moving battles of North Africa. In 1957 the University of Oxford, with the support of Lord Nuffield, established a fund for neurological research in Cairns' memory.

Webb-Johnson felt it was essential that the views of these new specialties should be heard in Council, but the existing system of election to Council could not ensure this. In 1944, Council decided to co-opt invited members from any specialty not represented by an elected member. Sir Henry Souttar (see also Fig 15.24) went further by suggesting that the College set up faculties in every specialty. This proved to be effective in the field of dental surgery and in anaesthetics, but was not extended to include other specialties at that stage, probably because the burgeoning specialty associations made such faculties largely unnecessary.

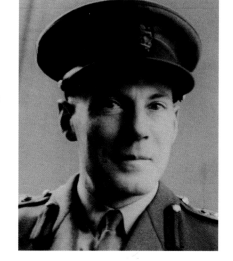

As always, surgery learnt from war, and many of the lessons were of direct importance in peace-time. One of these lessons is often given too little attention, namely the importance of good general health. One of the great differences between the First and Second World Wars was that troops in the latter were much more thoroughly prepared; they were fitter and 'harder', thanks to good food and strenuous training.

The blood transfusion service, which owed so much to the input of the College laboratories between the wars and to the work of Professor Beattie, was an extraordinary scheme based entirely on the voluntary donations of millions of citizens who would probably not otherwise have regarded themselves as particularly altruistic. Their only reward for a needle in the arm and the loss of a pint of blood was a cup of tea, a smile from the nurse, and a cheap enamel badge, which most donors were too shy to display.

By the end of the war, the army blood service could provide 40 litres of blood for every hundred casualties in front-line areas. With the coming of peace, a similarly lavish provision of blood made it possible to carry out surgical procedures that had hitherto been impossible. The study of the physiology of shock and blood transfusion led to a revolution in the management of major trauma and burns.

5.12 Sir Alexander Fleming (1881–1955)

Fleming trained at St Mary's Hospital and achieved the FRCS in 1909. After the First World War, he returned to St Mary's, where he taught bacteriology until his retirement as emeritus professor in 1948, although he continued as head of the Wright-Fleming Institute of Microbiology. Fleming discovered lysozyme in 1922 and in 1928, while engaged in research on *staphylococci*, discovered penicillin. Realising that crude penicillin was too weak as a therapeutic agent, he tried unsuccessfully to concentrate it. Sir Howard Florey and EB Chain at Oxford established penicillin as a therapeutic agent in 1943, and the three of them shared the Nobel Prize in Medicine in 1945.

(Courtesy Wellcome Institute Library, London)

5.12

In turn, towards the end of the war the concept of the 'golden hour' became ingrained – the need for early evacuation of the wounded soldier and the idea that intravenous fluid replacement should be started at the site of injury on the battlefield. This understanding was reinforced by the war in Korea, where improved transfusion equipment and helicopter evacuation improved survival. However, it was many years before this practice was applied to civilian injuries in Britain and victims of major road accidents were brought to hospital by helicopter.

The first primitive antimicrobial agents, the sulphonamides, were available in small quantities at the beginning of the war, but were ineffective against *staphylococci*. Towards the end of the war, Alexander Fleming's (Fig 5.12) chance discovery of penicillin was developed by Howard Florey, clinically tested by Hugh Cairns, and at first restricted to the armed forces. When penicillin became available to civilian surgeons, it transformed surgery once again. Perhaps even more important was the realisation that even more powerful antibiotics were waiting to be discovered in the natural world.

College Secretaries

Okey Belfour, *Secretary 1800–1811*

Having served as Clerk to the Company of Surgeons since 1782, Belfour oversaw the transition from the Company to the College. He was appointed Secretary in 1800 and helped draft the Charter of the new College.

Edmund Belfour, *Secretary 1811–1865*

Upon his father's retirement in 1811, Edmund Belfour took over as Secretary. The *Lancet* recorded that he was imbued with the conservative views of the older members of the Court of Assistants (later Council): 'He was opposed to the present plan of electing Councillors, being a strong supporter of self-election as the only means to secure respectability, although admitting that up to the present time the gentlemen elected were of as high character and ability as any who could have been admitted under the self-electing principle.'

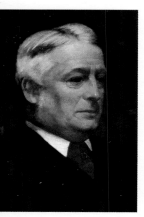

S1 Edward Trimmer
Secretary 1865–1901

Trimmer spent a period in the India Office before coming to the College as Assistant Secretary in 1859, when that office was first created. He was Co-Secretary of the committee during the complicated negotiations in 1872 to arrange an examination that should serve as 'one portal of entry' to the profession. He was also the first Secretary to the Committee of Management of the Conjoint Board from 1884 to 1887. He was a genial man with a strong personality and a remarkable memory for the contents of the College Charter and bylaws.

By Emily M Merrick

S2 Sibert Forrest Antrobus Cowell
Secretary 1901–1934

Cowell was Assistant Secretary from 1888 until he was appointed Secretary in 1901. Cowell was a quiet, reliable and conscientious man, and experienced the difficult times of the First World War and the more active years of Lord Moynihan's Presidency.

By Moussa Ayoub

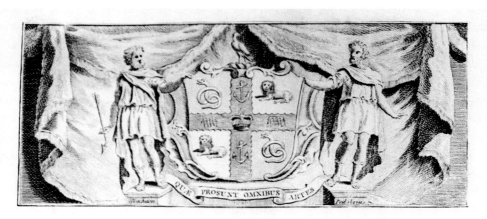

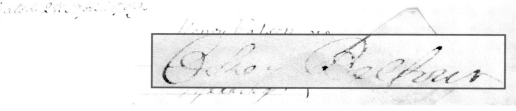

Until 1977 the College preserved an archaic distinction between College staff: they were either officers (senior members of the Scientific Departments, the Library, the General Department and the Examination Hall) or servants. When the Standing Rules were revised in that year, officers became 'senior staff' and the term 'servants' was abandoned. The College Secretary was identified as head of the General Department.

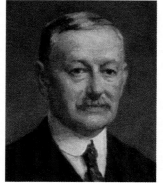

S2

The early Secretaries attended and took minutes of all meetings, boards and committees of the College as well as being in charge of junior staff. They wrote correspondence, sent out notices and

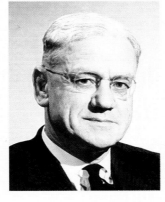

S3 Donald Kennedy Cassels
Secretary 1934–1962

Cassels came to the College in 1924 to help his uncle, Forrest Cowell, in the Secretary's Office. He was appointed Assistant Secretary in 1928 and succeeded Cowell in 1934. Cassels was also Secretary of the Imperial Cancer Research Fund from 1938 to 1960. He took an active administrative part in the post-war reconstruction of the College, its rebirth as a teaching centre and the expansion in the activities of the College initiated by Lord Webb-Johnson.

S4 Ronald Johnson-Gilbert
Secretary 1962–1988

Johnson-Gilbert served as Assistant Secretary from 1953 until his appointment as Secretary in 1962. He was responsible for the concept of the Hunterian Institute. He was also Secretary of the Joint Meeting of Surgical Colleges, the Joint Conference of Surgical Colleges, the International Federation of Surgical Colleges, the Joint Committee on Higher Surgical Training, the Faculty of Anaesthetists (until 1983) and the Faculty of Dental Surgery (until 1987).

S5 Roger Duffett
Secretary 1988–1997

Duffett came to the College in 1988 after 32 years with British Petroleum, and retired in 1997. Unlike his predecessors, Duffett had no previous experience of College affairs, although his grandfather was a Fellow and his father a Member of the College. His experience in industry had great advantages in what proved to be a decade of major upheaval.

S6 Craig Duncan, *Secretary 1997–*

Duncan came to the College in 1982 after working at the Universities of Durham and Southampton. He worked as Assistant Secretary of the Institute of Basic Medical Sciences, Secretary of the Hunterian Institute, Assistant Secretary of the College and Secretary for External Affairs before he became Secretary. This was a time when surgical politics, with which Duncan was very much at home, were becoming a major concern for the College.

S7 Craig Duncan and team, 1999

Back row (left to right): David Munn, Deputy College Secretary and Finance Board Secretary, Natalie Briggs, Education Board Secretary, Anne Bishop, Assistant College Secretary, Patricia Hagan, External Affairs Board Secretary, Martyn Coomer, Research Board Secretary.

Front row: Karen Smith, Training Board Secretary, Craig Duncan, College Secretary, Sarah Robinson, Examinations Board Secretary.

edicts of the College and arranged for publications. At times these functions included tasks as varied as arranging spectators and unrolling a mummy in the museum! In 1814 the salary was £200 per annum, and the Secretary lived in the College. In 1988 the role was still couched in archaic terms. Before a Secretary could be formally appointed, the President was required to read out the lengthy 'Summary of Duties', and the proleptic Secretary made the following declaration: 'I declare that I will be a good and faithful Secretary to The Royal College of Surgeons of England; that I will not, by any means, reveal any of the lawful Secrets thereof; and that I will duly, diligently, honestly and obediently perform the Duties of my Office, to the best of my knowledge and ability.'

S4

To those who have had no reason to think otherwise, the College has always been a single entity; the reality until the early 1990s was very different. A clause in the 1988 Regulations was revealing: 'The Secretary shall be responsible to the President and Council for the supervision and direction of all other members of the staff, except insofar as their duties may be under the supervision and direction of the Officers in Charge of the Scientific Departments, the Warden of Nuffield College or the Librarian.' Not only these departments but also the Court of Examiners and the Examinations Department, the Museums and the Teaching Departments all conducted themselves as separate entities.

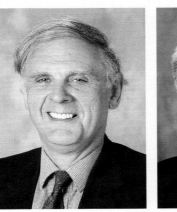

S5   S6

However, changes in the Charter and Ordinances in 1977 and 1987 and reorganisations that they enabled ensured that by 1992 the President, Council and the Secretary became responsible for the College as a single coherent entity. Since 1800 the many changes in the Charter, Ordinances, Standing Rules and Regulations have reflected changes in the governance of the College. Although their study is only of arcane interest, they reveal that the style of the College today is very different from that of two centuries ago. The College has had to adjust to the demands of the outside world.

S7

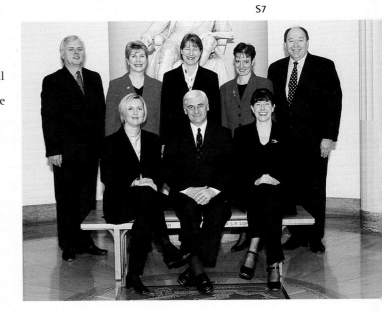

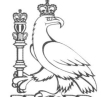

CHAPTER 6

After the Second World War: An Historic Recovery

6.1 Council of 1946

Left to right: Sir Hugh Cairns, Arthur Tudor Edwards, Sir James Paterson Ross, Sir Charles Max Page, Sir Ernest Frederick Finch, Lionel Edward Close Norbury, Sir Vincent Zachary Cope, Robert John McNeill Love, Sir Reginald Watson-Jones, Sir William Heneage Ogilvie (Vice-President), Arthur Henry Burgess, Lord Webb-Johnson (President), Sir Henry Sessions Souttar, Sir Cecil Wakeley (Vice-President), Sir Harry Platt, Sir Albert James Walton, Sir Geoffrey Langdon Keynes, Philip Henry Mitchiner, Julian Taylor, Lambert Charles Rogers, Robert Joseph Willan, George Grey Turner, Robert Paul Scott Mason, Sir Gordon Gordon-Taylor.

By Henry Carr

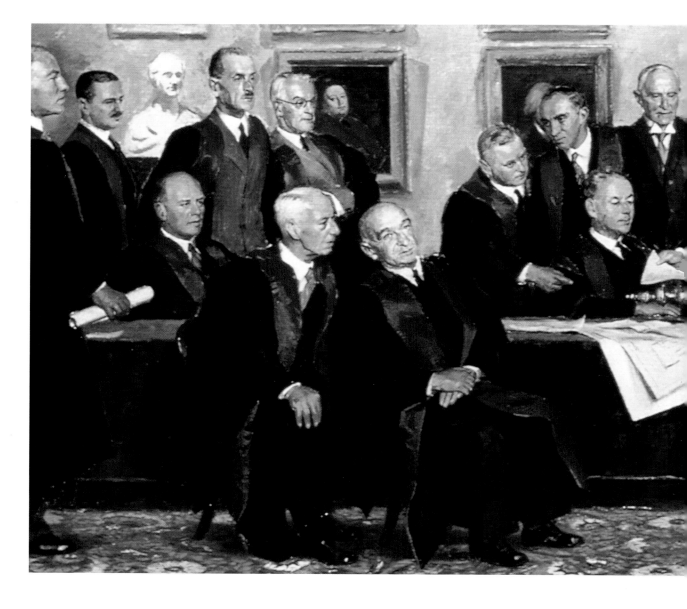

The group portrait of Council (Fig 6.1) commissioned shortly after the Second World War by the President Lord Webb-Johnson portrays a number of remarkable men, each of whom played a major role in surgical developments. Their skills and dedication were invaluable in shaping the future of the College and in addressing the many issues it faced at a time when its buildings lay in ruins.

Basic science courses had been offered throughout the war and were subsequently expanded into the Institute of Basic Sciences, greatly strengthening the College's scientific foundation. A training committee was formed in 1959. These two steps were part of a powerful post-war recovery that brought the College into one of the most active and stimulating periods of its history.

Rebuilding

The first task after the war was to rebuild the College premises (Fig 6.2). Begun in 1951, the re-building did not merely reconstruct what had been there before but included extensive additions.

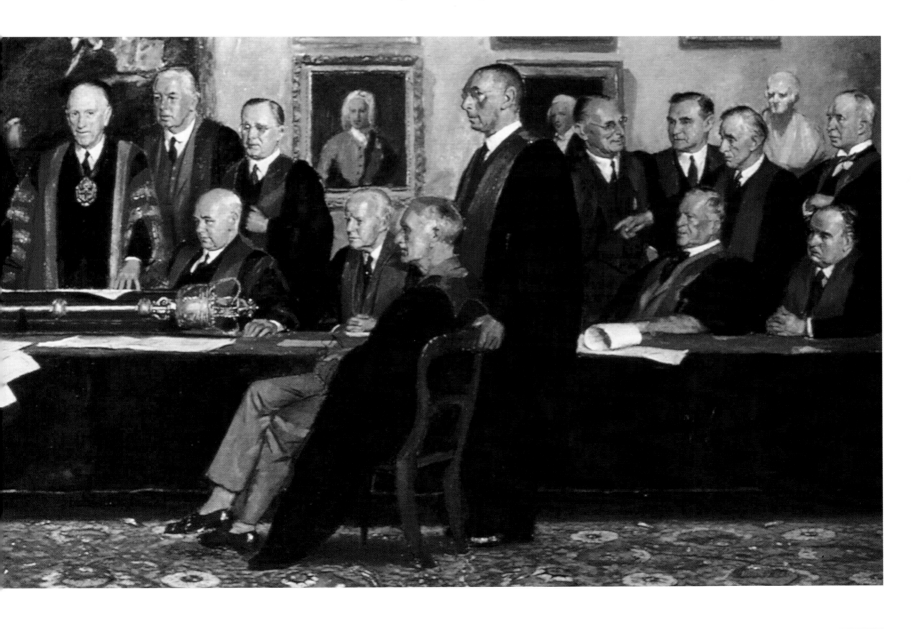

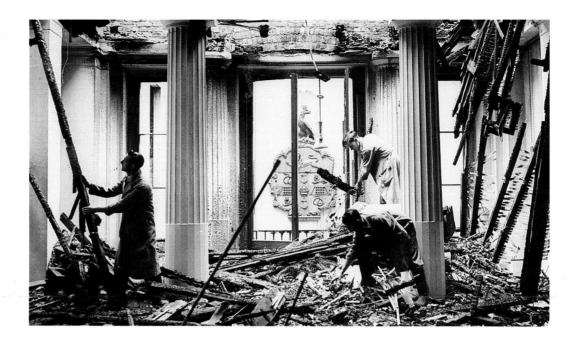

6.2 Sorting through the rubble left by a bomb in 1941

The building was modernised, open fires were removed and a gas-fired steam boiler was installed for central heating. Gas was piped to the new laboratories, and electric lifts were installed.

Gifts were received from sister organisations all over the world. Fellows gave named chairs for a new lecture theatre, and each member of Council provided one for the Council room. A generous donation from Ethicon Ltd panelled the Council room (Fig 6.3) in oak from a tree planted in the reign of Elizabeth I. In 1951 the College was given £75,000 by an anonymous benefactor later revealed as Edward Lumley (Fig 6.4). His generosity made it possible to incorporate into the new building a magnificent lecture hall, which was named after him (Fig 6.5).

The death of Sir John Bland-Sutton's widow in 1943 gave rise to a dispute over Sir John's estate, which in turn brought into question the charitable status of the College. As the result

6.3 The Council Room

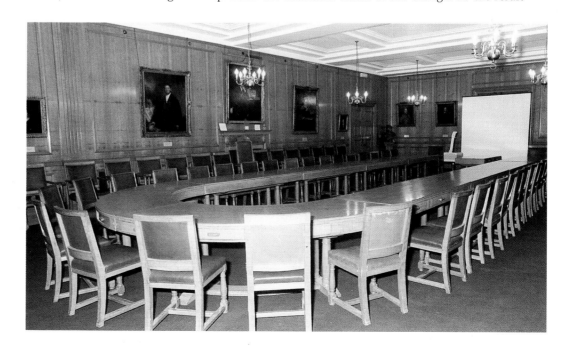

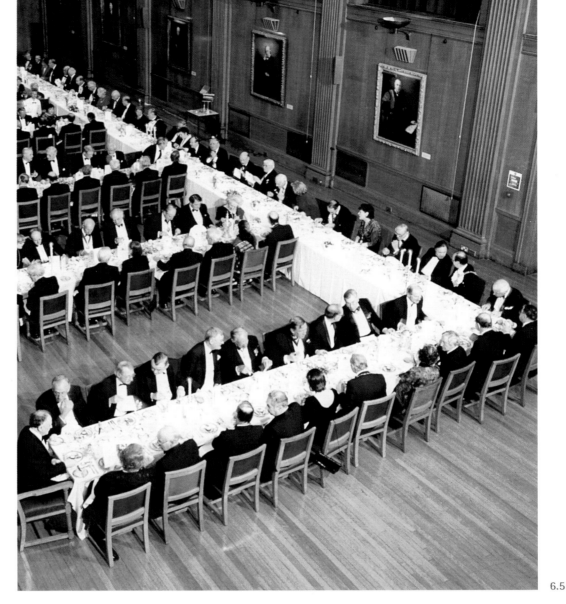

6.5

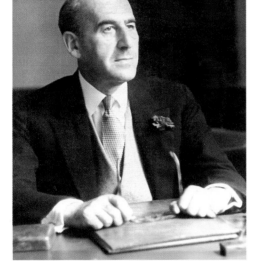

6.4 Edward Lumley (1892–1960)

Originally from Melbourne, Edward Lumley came to London as a boy and became an insurance broker with his father. After service in France in the Great War, he returned to Australia to establish companies to sell Lloyd's insurance across the country and in New Zealand. His interest in the College arose through an introduction to Sir Reginald Watson-Jones. He also endowed a fellowship with the Australasian College to assist surgeons to research in the UK.

(Courtesy of Mr Henry Lumley)

6.5 The Edward Lumley Hall

of an appeal to the House of Lords, the charitable status of the College, with its attendant tax advantages, was clearly defined. From then on, as a Registered Charity, the College could appeal for legacies and donations. This clarification was timely, for post-war inflation had escalated the costs of rebuilding, and five years into the rebuilding programme the lack of funding became a serious handicap.

At the end of 1956 Sir Archibald McIndoe warned Council that rebuilding would have to stop unless another £200,000 could be found at once. In the words of Sir Harry Platt:

> I remember Council made a contract with the builders such that the bomb-damaged College would be rebuilt, but if the money ran out, there was a "stop clause" – the roof would be made weatherproof but all other work would stop. I used to go to Baker Street for luncheon with Simon Marks. Price Thomas was usually too busy so Archibald McIndoe came.

One day after luncheon, over coffee, I mentioned to Simon Marks that the cash flow was drying up. He gave no sign that he had heard or understood. When Archie and I were outside, Archie said, "Harry, he said nothing!" Two weeks later we had luncheon again with Simon. I told him that we had activated the "stop" clause. "You've stopped the rebuilding?" We explained that there was no alternative. "Start again," said Simon, "and do not worry about paying the bills." Soon afterwards we had his cheque for £750,000 from a family trust. The rebuilding went ahead.

6.6 Lord Marks (1888–1964)

At the age of 18, Simon Marks went into the business his father had founded in penny bazaar stores in Leeds. After the First World War, he expanded the Marks & Spencer chain of stores throughout the country. He gave generously to the College. This photograph shows Marks receiving an Honorary Fellowship of the College from Sir Harry Platt.

This episode led to the formation in 1958 of an Appeal Committee with Lord Kindersley (Chairman of Lazard Brothers) as Chairman, Sir Simon Marks (Fig 6.6) as Vice-Chairman, and William Davis as Appeal Secretary. The opening event was a screening of the film *Life in Emergency Ward 10* in the Edward Lumley Hall. For the first time, annual subscriptions were requested from old Fellows

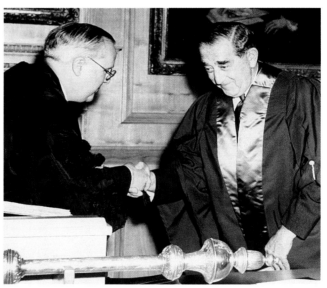

6.6

and required of all new ones. Over the next 13 years £3.8 million was collected, including a magnificent bequest from the McRae-Webb-Johnson Fund.

6.7 Floor plan of the ground level of The Royal College of Surgeons, 1959

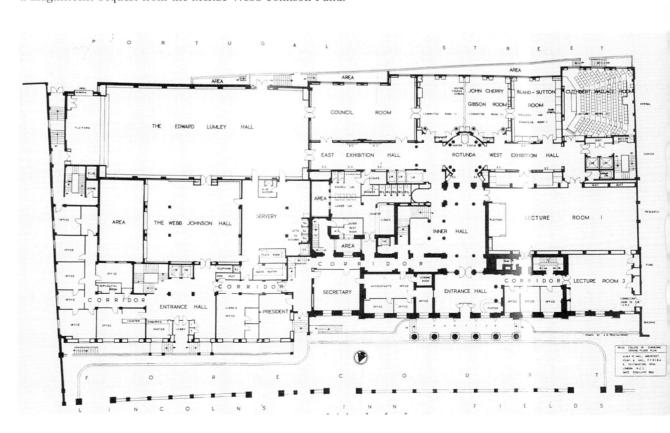

The first phase of the rebuilding – completed in 1959 (Fig 6.7) – included the laboratories for the Departments of Anatomy, Pathology, Dental Science and Research in Ophthalmology, three demonstration rooms, the Odontological Museum, the Animal House, the Cuthbert Wallace Lecture Room, the Fellows' and Examiners' Room, two new Committee rooms, the Rotunda and West Exhibition Hall and the Howard Gray Library. Reconstruction of the west wing of the main College building, additional space for the Departments of Anatomy and Physiology, new laboratories for the Department of Pharmacology, office accommodation for the Joint Secretariat for Specialist Associations, the Library Rare Book Room, and two more ground floor lecture rooms were completed in 1962.

Her Majesty The Queen and His Royal Highness The Duke of Edinburgh visited the College on 7 November 1962, formally opened the newest part of the building and inspected the completely restored College. This visit is commemorated by a silver plaque above the chimney-piece in the inner hall. The Prime Minister, the Rt Hon Harold Macmillan, opened the new Hunterian Museum on 17 May 1963, marking the 150th anniversary of the original opening of the Hunterian Collection in 1813.

Nuffield College of Surgical Sciences

In addition to its traditional role of an examining body and its newer research activities, the College emerged from the war as a teaching centre. The courses in basic sciences attracted surgeons from all over the world, many of them fresh from the armed services and eager to obtain the Fellowship diploma. In those days it was difficult to find accommodation of any kind in London, which was pockmarked with bomb sites and where rented flats were largely in the hands of racketeers.

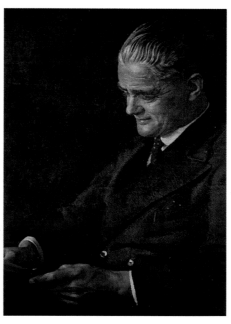

6.8

6.8 Lord Nuffield (1877–1963)

William Morris started by repairing bicycles, then ran his own garage, and ended up as a millionaire motor manufacturer (Morris Minors are still popular among restorers, and Nuffield's initials live on in the 'MG', which stands for Morris Garages). Interested since childhood in surgical sciences, Nuffield became a generous donor to innumerable medical institutions and a good friend of the College. In 1942 he was awarded the Honorary Medal of the College for services to British medicine.

By John Wheatley ARA, 1950

In February 1948, Council decided to convert the houses next door into temporary accommodation for postgraduate students, trusting that somehow the money would be found. Sir Hugh Cairns (see also Fig 5.11) had been a friend of Lord Nuffield (Fig 6.8) since his undergraduate days, and Nuffield had recently funded his professorial unit at Oxford. Now, at the urging of Cairns, Nuffield provided the money for the conversion of 44 and 45 Lincoln's Inn Fields. In 1949 the first residents – including students from Australia, Canada, South Africa, United States, China, India and Ireland – moved in, with Ray Last as Warden. Lord Nuffield followed this benefaction with an additional gift of £250,000 to start building the Nuffield College of Surgical Sciences, a grand name for a postgraduate hostel.

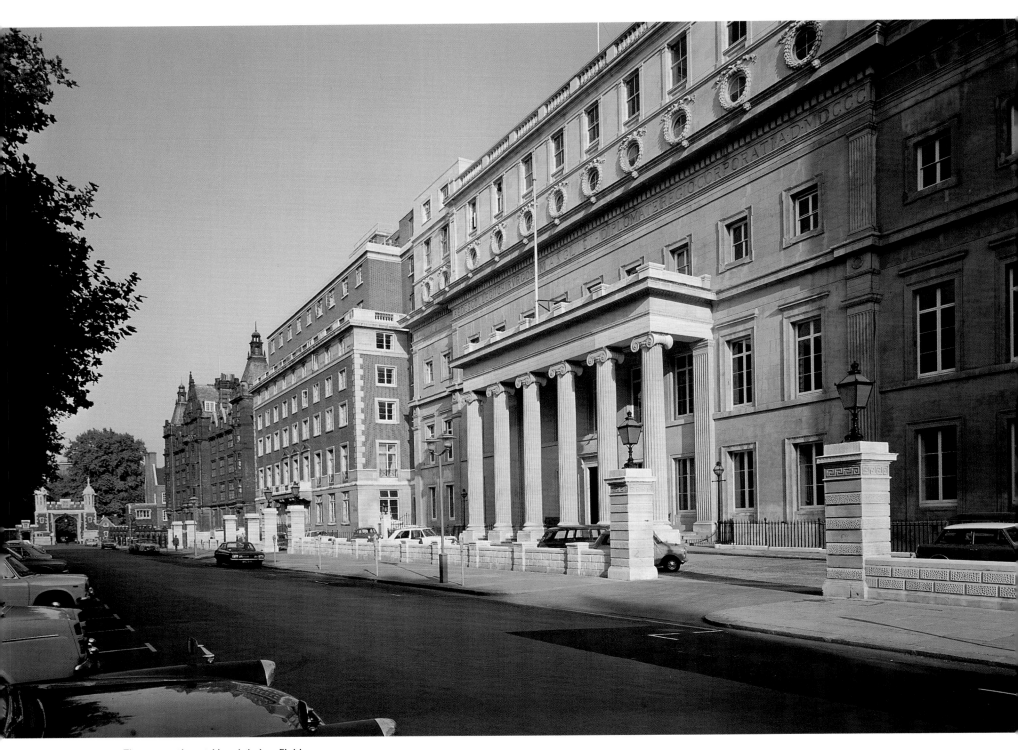

6.9 The properties at Lincoln's Inn Fields:
the Nuffield College of Surgical Sciences
on the left, the main College building
on the right, c. 1959

A supplemental grant of £175,000 from King Edward's Hospital Fund for London made it possible to complete construction of Nuffield College in 1957. On the 5th of April Lord Freyberg VC, a close friend of Lord Nuffield, ceremoniously opened the door between the Edward Lumley and Webb-Johnson halls. The new College provided 80 residential units plus the President's Lodge, a squash court, a billiard room, a common room, writing and reading rooms, a dining room and administrative offices (Fig 6.9).

This was the heyday of Nuffield College. It was full of men from throughout the Commonwealth who worked hard, played hard and made full use of the bar (Fig 6.10) where the noise in the evening often matched that of the builders during the day. The College courses in basic sciences were always over-subscribed, and two of the most popular teachers – David Slome and Frank Stansfield – offered intensive evening classes at a nominal fee (Fig 6.11).

6.10 Students in the Nuffield bar in 1954

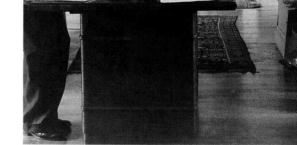

6.10

The Institute of Basic Medical Sciences

As its regular courses were expensive to run, the College sought external help. At the time, the University Grants Committee would only support units that were part of a university. It was proposed to overcome this difficulty by a merger with the British Postgraduate Medical Federation (BPMF), which was affiliated with the University of London. Despite the misgivings of Lord Webb-Johnson, who believed that the College should remain independent of any outside body, the merger went ahead; by 1950 the College courses were organised into a new Institute of Basic Medical Sciences within the BPMF,

6.11 Professor David Slome teaching

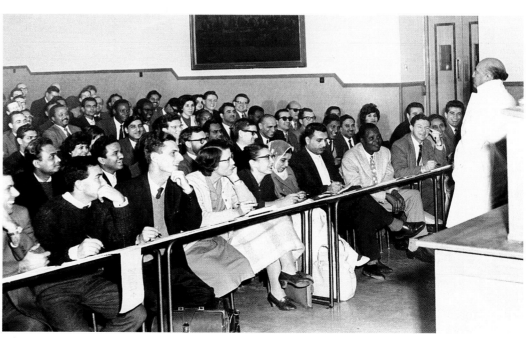

6.11

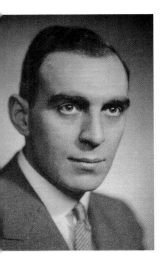

6.12 Sir Reginald Watson-Jones (1902–1972)

Watson-Jones was a brilliant orthopaedic surgeon and the first director of the orthopaedic and accident department at the London Hospital. He founded the *Journal of Bone and Joint Surgery*, and also wrote *Fractures and Joint Injuries*, one of the most popular textbooks ever. The annual Watson-Jones Lecture is endowed in his memory.

6.13 The centenary of ether anaesthesia, October 1946

HRH The Princess Royal unveiling a commemorative plaque in the College with Lord Webb-Johnson.

6.14 Sir Roy Yorke Calne (b. 1930)

After qualifying from Guy's Hospital, Calne demonstrated anatomy at Oxford and received his surgical training at the Royal Free and St Mary's Hospitals, London, and the Peter Bent Brigham Hospital in Boston. He was appointed Senior Lecturer at the Westminster Hospital and became Professor of Surgery at the University of Cambridge. Calne has made seminal contributions to the field of transplant immunology, and his honours include Fellowship to the Royal Society. Calne is a skilled artist. At the College he won the Hallet and Jacksonian prizes, was awarded a Hunterian Professorship and delivered the 1989 Hunterian Oration. He was a Council member from 1981 to 1990 and Vice-President from 1986 to 1989.

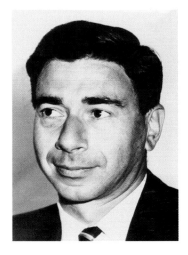

with Sir Reginald Watson-Jones (Fig 6.12) as its first Chairman. In the plans for the new College, the Institute was assigned spacious accommodation in the southern part of the building. Teaching and research museums in anatomy and pathology were generously provided by the Wellcome Trust.

The Departments of Anatomy, Physiology and Pathology were incorporated into the new Institute. Pharmacology joined in 1954 but was housed in the Examination Hall, Queen Square, until 1962. With the establishment of a Chair in 1963, Biochemistry separated from Physiology and was joined by the Department of Biophysics in 1983. The research activities of the Institute attracted considerable charitable monies, notably the James Cotton Chair of Biochemistry, the Rank Chair in Biophysics, ICI support and subsequently the Vandervell Chair in Pharmacology.

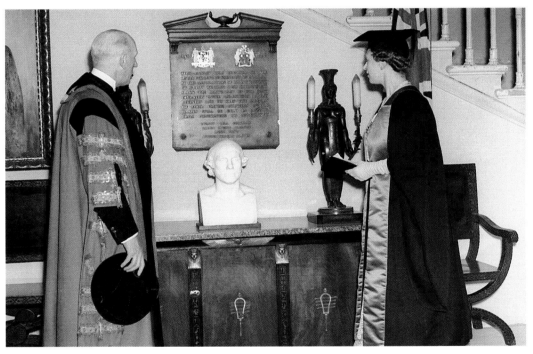

6.13

The research output from these departments was considerable and gained world-wide recognition. Pharmacology in particular fostered three Fellows of the Royal Society and a Nobel Prize winner in Sir John Vane. The Faculties of Anaesthetists and Dental Surgery ran their own distinguished research units within the College (Fig 6.13). The Buckston Browne Research Farm at Downe had been donated to the College in 1933. In 1949 Council recommended its closure in view of its isolated position and lack of multi-disciplinary activities. The recommendation included the transfer of experimental work on large animals to a more conveniently situated laboratory such as the Royal Veterinary School. However, the immediate past President, Sir Hugh Lett (Buckston Browne's son-in-law), delivered a powerful letter of opposition to Council. Council withdrew its recommendation and Professor Slome, head of the Physiology Department, took over responsibility for the farm in 1951; this continued for a further 25 years. Research included some basic studies in the field of transplantation, first by William Dempster, and later by Sir Roy Calne (Fig 6.14).

6.15 Lord Brock (1903–1980)

After studying at Guy's Medical School, Russell Brock became Hunterian Professor in 1928. In 1929 he was awarded a Rockefeller Travelling Fellowship and went to St Louis, from which time he developed his interest in thoracic surgery. During the war he was thoracic surgeon and regional adviser in thoracic surgery to the EMS. He was a pioneer in numerous cardio-thoracic techniques and served as President of both the Thoracic Society and the Society of Cardiovascular Surgeons of Great Britain and Ireland. He was elected to Council in 1949 and was President from 1963 to 1966. On retirement from his surgical posts he was the first and only director of the College's Department of Surgical Sciences, as well as a member of the Court of Patrons and Chairman of the Hunterian Trustees. Out of Brock's interest in history grew his involvement in restoring the old operating theatre of St Thomas's Hospital.

By Carlos Sancha

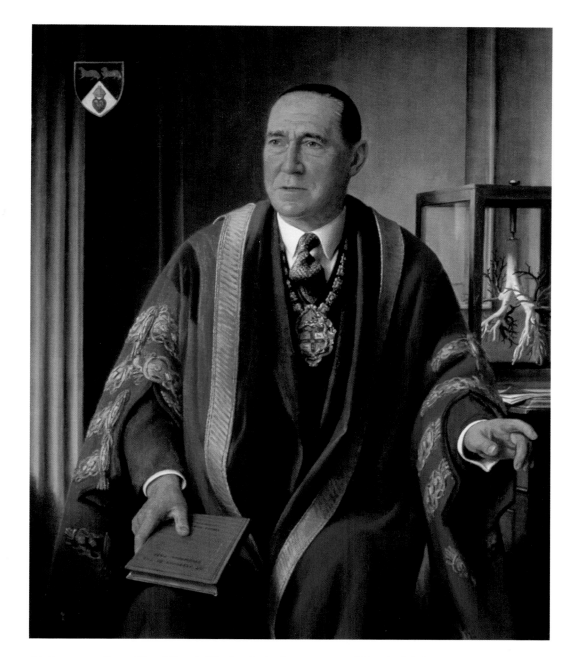

At the suggestion of Lord Brock (Fig 6.15), the Department of Surgical Science was set up in 1968 with sponsorship from the Freemasons' 250th Anniversary Fund, the Medical Research Council and the British Heart Foundation. In 1975, when Lord Brock retired as its first Director, the Department was merged with that of Physiology.

The Hunterian Institute

By 1979, as Lord Webb-Johnson had predicted, relations between the Institute of Basic Medical Sciences and the College came under strain. The Institute cost about £800,000 per annum, only half of which was provided by the University of London. The College supplied valuable space, heating and lighting as well as some £75,000 per annum. The rest came from research grants won by the various members of the Institute. The College gained prestige from their publications, and the research facilities attracted basic science teachers of the highest quality, but the financial foundations of the Institute were insecure.

The University of London had become alarmed at the disproportionate cost of medicine in the University; as a result, a working party on medical and dental teaching resources was set up under Lord Flowers to cut costs. The *Flowers Report* was published in 1980. The working party had inspected every postgraduate institute in London and ranked them according to the quality and quantity of their research; those that fell below a designated line were to have their grant phased out over the next four years. The Institute of Basic Medical Sciences fell well below this line.

The College Secretary, Ronald Johnson-Gilbert, warned Council that the College on its own could not fund the Institute of Basic Sciences. The grant was to cease in 1984. Three years later the Department of Health also withdrew its funding from dental research into a vaccine against caries that was being carried out at the Buckston Browne Farm.

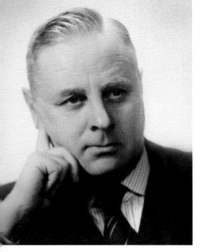
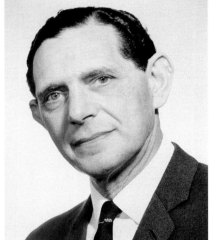

6.16   6.17

In 1985 Council decided to continue supporting the Institute for five more years, albeit under a new name: the Institute of Basic Medical Sciences became the Hunterian Institute of Surgical Education and Sciences. Sir Gordon Robson (see also Fig 12.14) was its first Master and Craig Duncan its Secretary. Lord Leverhulme responded with characteristic generosity to an appeal for funding, and there followed an endowment from the Rank Foundation to support a new Department of Physics, under David Gadian, in the exciting new field of nuclear magnetic resonance.

6.16 Robert McNeill Love (1891–1974)

Co-author with Hamilton Bailey of the famous under-graduate textbook, *Short Practice of Surgery*, he ran a famous FRCS course at the Royal Northern Hospital.

6.17 Alan Apley (1914–1996)

Apley started his internationally renowned orthopaedic course at the Rowley Bristow Hospital, Pyrford in 1948, with the motto 'listen, look, feel, move; then X-ray'. His lecture notes were published as the *System of Orthopaedics and Fractures*, published in its seventh edition in 1995. In 1973 he was elected to Council and became Vice-President. He also served as President of the Orthopaedic Section of the Royal Society of Medicine, President of the British Orthopaedic Association and editor of the *Journal of Bone and Joint Surgery*.

The demand for more courses continued, as did the drain on the College's finances. In 1988 Sir Stanley Peart was invited to be the new Master of the Hunterian Institute. His task became impossible: to maintain in-house research of high quality while reducing expenditure. The challenge was not helped by a new generation of surgeons on Council who believed that the main activity of the College should be the education and training of surgeons, and that surgical research was more appropriately undertaken in university departments of surgery in the hospitals where surgery was actually performed. The Buckston Browne Farm seemed to many to be as outdated as it was isolated. The balance had been lost between the ivory tower pursuit of fundamental research, and teaching trainees the basics of their profession. Many believed that much of what went on in the College, and consumed so much of its money, had little relevance to surgery.

There were passionate debates. It was difficult for some to accept that the activities of the College had changed – it was no longer the only centre of surgical research in the British Isles and it was having difficulty keeping up with the increasing demands for training in the new surgical technologies. Nevertheless, senior figures who had given so much to revive the College after the Second World War now warned that donations to the College would dry up if research ceased to be undertaken in-house.

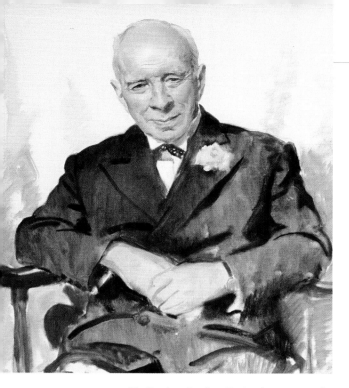

6.18 Sir Gordon Gordon-Taylor (1878–1960)

Famous for his technical skill in hind-quarter amputation, he was an enthusiastic examiner, and a kind and encouraging mentor to Australasians visiting London to study for the FRCS. In 1934, he participated in the second Primary examination held in Australia, and examined five further times there, as well as in Calcutta and Colombo. In 1949 the Australasian College founded the Gordon-Taylor prize in his honour for the best candidate in their Primary examination. In 1950, he was appointed Sub-Dean of the Institute of Basic Medical Sciences in recognition of his assistance to overseas students.

By Sir James Gunn, 1960

6.19 Lord Smith (1914–1998)

A man of diverse interests, from music to painting to cricket, Rodney Smith was known especially for his diplomatic skills and ability to resolve political conflicts affecting the medical profession. Trained at St Thomas's, in 1939 Smith was appointed surgical registrar at the Middlesex Hospital, where he became acquainted with Lord Webb-Johnson, who helped steer his attention towards the College. During the Second World War, Smith served in the Royal Army Medical Corps. Afterwards, he was appointed consultant surgeon to St George's Hospital which he turned into Britain's leading centre for treatment of biliary and pancreatic disorders. Through-out his career, Smith was active in the life of the College, having served on the Court of Examiners and Council, as well as being Dean of the Institute of Basic Medical Sciences before becoming President in 1973.

By GJD Bruce

In 1991 Council set up a working party under the chairmanship of Sir Michael Peckham to report on 'future policy for surgical education and research'. The working party reported in February 1992 and strongly supported the commitment of the College to surgical education and research, but not necessarily all in-house. They recommended the establishment of a Department of Surgical Education and the introduction of a research fellowship scheme for surgeons-in-training (see also Chapter 11), along with closure of the Hunterian Institute. Council accepted the report and the need to end in-house surgical research.

Surgical Training

Three years after the war, the National Health Service (NHS) was inaugurated. Peripheral hospitals, with the exception of the temporary prefabricated sector hospitals that had been hastily constructed at the beginning of the war, had long been neglected. Many of the peripheral hospitals were Poor Law institutions that had never had a surgeon with an FRCS on the staff. The new NHS was faced with a huge need for surgeons.

To meet this demand, the College responded by sponsoring clinical courses for the Final FRCS in addition to their basic science commitment. New courses sprang up all over the country. Perhaps the most famous were those at the Royal Northern Hospital run by Robert McNeill Love (Fig 6.16), at the Royal Marsden by Ronald Raven (see also Fig 8.3), and at Pyrford (in orthopaedics) by Alan Apley (Fig 6.17).

6.19

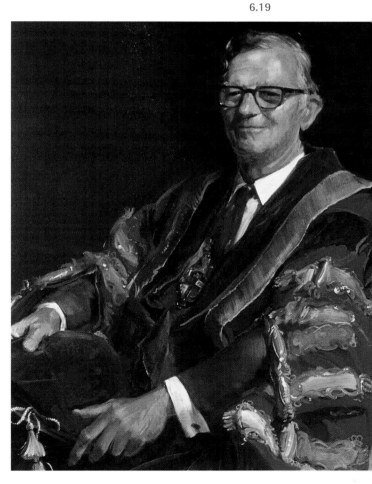

As the number of these courses grew, so did the need for someone to co-ordinate them and to guide trainees in their studies for the FRCS. For young surgeons from the Commonwealth, Sir Gordon Gordon-Taylor (Fig 6.18) acted as unofficial counsellor and confidant upon whom new arrivals did well to call at the earliest opportunity. His example made it clear that every young surgeon, not only those from overseas, needed a mentor.

In 1957 Mrs V Penrose May provided an endowment for a surgical tutor who would have the task of advising postgraduate students in the College. Rodney Smith (Fig 6.19) became the first Penrose May Tutor. By 1960, he was running full-time courses for two batches of 16 postgraduates each year, involving more than 30 hospitals and hundreds of consultants.

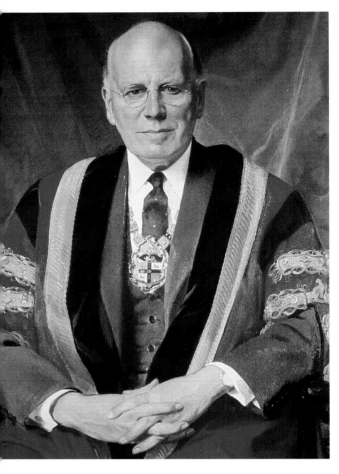

6.20 Professor Sir James Paterson Ross (1895–1980)

Pupil of Harvey Cushing and private assistant to Lord Moynihan, he became Professor of Surgery at St Bartholomew's Hospital in 1935 and was famous for performing a lumbar sympathectomy on King George VI, thereby saving his leg. He served as President of the College from 1957–1960, and then became Director of the British Postgraduate Medical Federation until 1966.

By James Gunn

The Hospital Recognition Committee

Inspection of training posts had begun in a small way before the war, but the visits were at ten-year intervals, and teaching hospitals were excused from inspection. With the inauguration of the NHS, the College insisted that candidates for the FRCS must have at least six months' experience in a casualty (accident and emergency) department. As casualty officers often received little training, they resented being exploited to man these key posts in the new NHS. This presented the College with an obligation to inspect casualty as well as surgical posts.

The Hospital Recognition Committee gradually became more influential. In 1967 visits became quinquennial and involved every member of Council. Visiting teams were charged to find out whether trainees received the right kind of surgical experience, who their teachers were, and what (if any) teaching was provided. The visitors inspected operating theatre records and were unimpressed by long lists of operations undertaken by trainees without senior supervision. They interviewed trainees alone. They insisted on seeing the living quarters and asked what (if any) food was available in the middle of the night when so much emergency surgery was done. Visits soon became formalised with a checklist and a detailed report to the Committee.

The Hospital Recognition Committee could recommend to Council the immediate withdrawal of recognition. In practice, hospitals were usually given six months to redress any weaknesses identified by the Committee before being re-checked. All four surgical Royal Colleges agreed on the list of posts approved for training; if approval was withdrawn, a hospital quickly found itself unable to recruit juniors for any surgical disciplines. Thus, the College had found its teeth: since every member of Council took part in these inspections, they provided a useful link with Fellows across the country and brought valuable feedback to the College.

The Training Committee

In 1959 Council established a Committee on the Training of Surgeons with wide terms of reference to consider surgical training and the Fellowship examination. Its membership included Sir James Paterson Ross, President (Fig 6.20), and Sir Archibald McIndoe (see also Fig 15.19) and Arthur Dickson Wright, Vice-Presidents. One might expect this group to represent the old guard in a reputedly conservative College. Quite the reverse: they began with explosive vigour and the reforms they sparked off took the next 40 years to implement. The group portrait of Council in 1960 (Fig 6.21) includes these unlikely revolutionaries.

The Committee produced ten interim reports. The first recommended that the granting of the Fellowship should be delayed until the end of training, but this was too radical for Council. Council was, however, more receptive to recommendations on a regional network of advisers and tutors, the length of training, reciprocity with the Royal Australasian College, and criteria for hospital recognition. The proposals also led to links with the specialist associations and

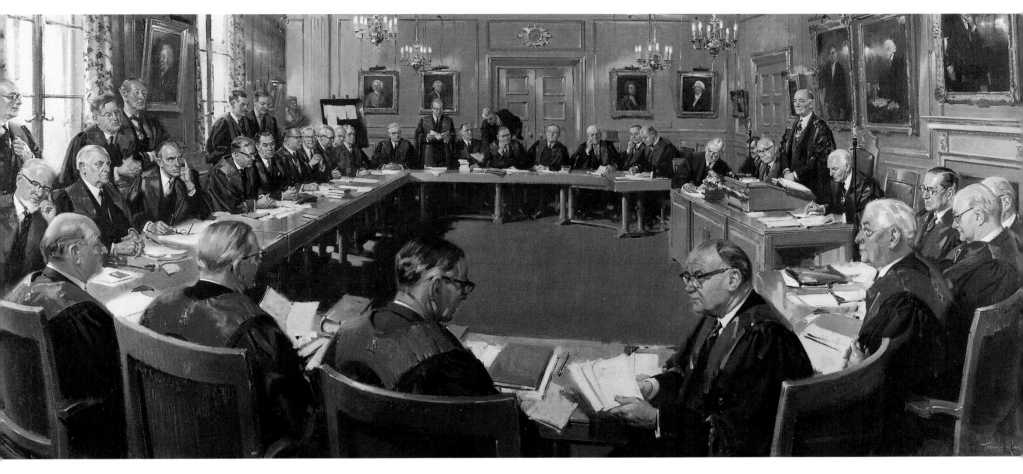

6.21 Council of 1960

Clockwise from the President, Lord Porritt: Professor Digby Chamberlain (Vice-President), Lord Brock, Julian Taylor, Sir Eric William Riches, Sir Clifford Naunton Morgan, Professor Charles Alexander Wells, Professor Ian Aird, Harold Clifford Edwards, Sir Thomas Holmes Sellors, Sir Henry Osmond-Clarke, Sir Frank Wild Holdsworth, Chapple Gill-Carey, Norman Leslie Capener, Geoffrey Stephen William Organe, Sir Reginald Watson-Jones, Humphrey George Edgar Arthure, Professor Martin Amsler Rushton, Professor David Waldron Smithers, Sir Edward Grainger Muir, Thomas Keith Selfe Lyle, John Henderson Hunt, Professor Leslie Norman Pyrah, Robert Victor Cooke, John Cridland Barrett, Professor Francis Roland Stammers, Ronald Henry Ottywell Betham Robinson, Professor Robert Milnes Walker, Ronald Stuart Johnson-Gilbert (Assistant Secretary), Sir Hedley John Barnard Atkins, Sir Clement Price Thomas, Arthur Dickson Wright, Lawrence Abel, Professor Sir James Paterson Ross, Kennedy Cassels (Secretary), William Frederick Davis (Deputy Secretary), Sir Stanford Cade (Vice-President).

By Terence Cuneo

the establishment of the Specialist Advisory Committees. Another radical proposal was the appointment of a professor of surgery at the College. This gained Council support, but no suitable applicant was identified. Subsequent debate modified the proposal to the development of a Department of Surgical Science.

Advisers and Tutors

The purpose of the 1960 recommendation of the Training Committee to set up a nation-wide network of regional advisers and tutors was to guide and assist young trainees. The Nuffield Provincial Hospitals Trust financed the pilot scheme, and the new College advisers and tutors threw themselves into the work with enthusiasm; they declined honoraria, preferring to use the Nuffield money to get the scheme up and running. The scheme was at once perceived to be a success and the College hailed as a pathfinder. There are now more than 250 College tutors in England and Wales, and one adviser in every region for each of the major specialties.

Specialist Advisory Committees

From the beginning, the Training Committee realised that it was necessary to identify posts that would be suitable for post-Fellowship training and, to do this, they needed advice from the specialist associations. The specialist associations were thinking along similar lines, and by 1966 specialist advisory committees (SACs) were established in each specialty, with representatives from all four surgical Royal Colleges and the relevant specialist association. A Joint Committee

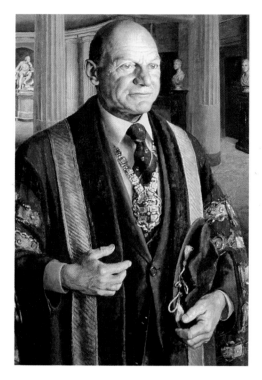

6.22 Sir Reginald Murley (1916–1997)

After serving in the Second World War attached to a field ambulance unit, Murley became a Fellow in 1946. He was appointed consultant general surgeon to the Royal Northern and City of St Albans Hospitals. His medical interests included the problems of thrombosis and the thyroid, as well as advocating conservative surgery for breast cancer. A strong opponent of nationalised medicine, he was a staunch supporter of the Fellowship for Freedom in Medicine. He was one of the first surgical tutors in the early 1960s, a regional adviser in 1965, was elected to Council in 1970 and served as President from 1977 to 1980. His life-long admiration for John Hunter culminated in his appointment as Chairman of the Hunterian Trustees in 1988.

By John Walton

on Higher Surgical Training was formed to bring these bodies together. The remit of the SACs was first to ensure that specialist registrars were receiving appropriate training, and secondly that there were approximately the right number of men and women in training to fill forecasted NHS consultant vacancies. The first specialties to put their houses in order were the orthopaedic and plastic surgeons; they were soon followed by others, reflecting the growing influence of the specialist associations in surgical practice in the United Kingdom (see also Chapter 15).

Reform of the FRCS Examination

In 1960, at its second meeting, the Training Committee turned its energy to the paradox whereby the FRCS – the highest diploma the College could confer – was accorded to a surgeon long before the completion of training. The Committee suggested that 'some means should be found of deferring the grant of the title of Fellow until a time when the candidate had fully completed his pre-consultant surgical training'. This initiative was in fact years ahead of its time, and Council rejected the report. However, the idea that the FRCS should come at the end, rather than at the beginning, of training would not go away. In spite of resistance both in and out of Council, the change was finally implemented in 1990 (see also Chapter 10).

The National Health Service

The concept of a national health service had been formulated in the 1930s, and even in the early years of the war, the Colleges were aware that hospitals could never go back to the pre-war system. The Medical Planning Commission, set up by the British Medical Association (BMA) in August 1940, included representatives from the three English Royal Colleges (The Royal College of Physicians, The Royal College of Surgeons and The Royal College of Obstetricians and Gynaecologists). The Colleges were not satisfied that the BMA could adequately represent the interests of consultants, as they considered the association to be politically motivated. Accordingly, they created their own Standing Joint Committee to consult directly with the government. The Colleges authorised the Committee to take executive action.

The period from December 1946, when the NHS Bill became law, to 5 July 1948, the 'appointed day' when the NHS came into existence, was a time of bitter opposition by doctors, led by the BMA. Although the three Presidents supported the Bill, there was considerable dissent within each College. There were many who saw any form of central planning as a threat to the freedom of the profession.

The main issue dividing the profession was whether or not to negotiate with the Minister of Health on the Regulations made under the Act. An extraordinary meeting of Council was called in November 1946 to consider the matter of negotiation, followed by a meeting of the Fellows. Council was in favour of negotiating but the Fellows were against it. The President did not allow a vote at the Fellows' meeting since no formal resolution had been circulated with the notice.

The three Presidents wrote to Aneurin Bevan on 2 January 1947, assuring him of their support for further negotiation but pointing out the fear that entering discussions would imply approval and acceptance of the main provisions of the Act. They asked the Minister for a statement on three contentious issues: remuneration; the mechanism for appeal against expulsion from the service; and interference with the liberty of movement of general practitioners. Bevan assured them that entering into discussions would not compromise their position.

The battle was not over. A group of 33 Fellows demanded an extraordinary meeting. They included Sir Reginald Murley (Fig 6.22), who went on to become President of the College, and FJ Gillingham, future President of the Royal College of Surgeons of Edinburgh. This meeting did take place in April 1948, and harsh words were spoken; but unlike the occasion in 1831 when Wakley was forcibly ejected from the lecture theatre, no violence occurred.

In retrospect it is clear that throughout the 1940s, Council, whatever the views of its individual members, was always willing to co-operate with government and had no wish to become involved in political turmoil. Surprisingly, the Bill received no coverage in the *Annals of the College*, which began publication in 1947.

6.23 The early post-war College Presidents

Left to right: Harry Platt, James Paterson Ross, Thomas Holmes Sellors, Arthur Porritt, Hedley Atkins, Cecil Wakeley, Russell Brock.

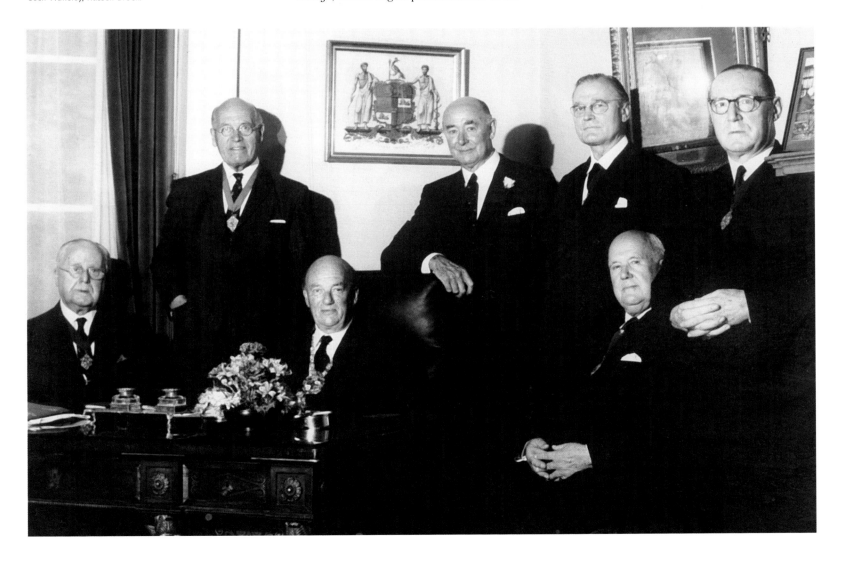

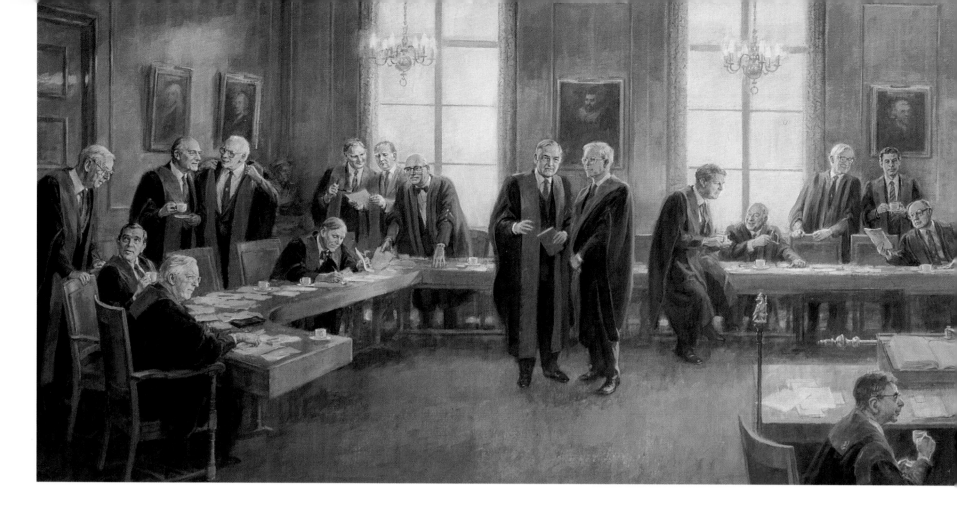

Post-war College governance

In 1953 Council consisted of 24 elected and seven co-opted members, the latter representing the
Faculties of Dental Surgery and Anaesthetists, and the specialties of general practice, obstetrics
and gynaecology, ophthalmology, otolaryngology and radiology. Representation of the Faculties
was enhanced by the 1967 Charter, when their Deans became ex-officio members of Council.
The 1977 supplemental charter and accompanying ordinances allowed for three elected Council
members, with full privileges, from each Faculty. The President and two Vice-Presidents were,
and still are, elected annually by Council, their term of office normally being three years for
President and two years for Vice-President (Fig 6.23). The 1972 Charter reduced Council tenure
from eight years with a further eight years if re-elected, to eight- and four-year terms, and
the candidate's age and date of Fellowship were added to the electoral information. The 1977
Charter also opened the election to all Fellows; previously, Fellows could not stand for an
election until they had held the Diploma for ten years.

The Diplomates ceremony was introduced in 1958 during the presidency of Sir James Paterson
Ross. The colourful regalia of President, Council and Diplomates during these events ensure a
memorable occasion for all those present. The ceremony is also a time for admitting Honorary
Fellows and presenting other College awards.

Living Honorary Fellows are restricted to 150, and the number of medically qualified Fellows
must not exceed 120. Non-medical Honorary Fellows include members of the Royal Family.
The Queen was elected in 1951 when she was Princess Elizabeth, The Queen Mother in 1950,
The Duke of Edinburgh in 1953, Princess Margaret in 1963, The Prince of Wales in 1976 and
The Princess Royal in 1986. Others elected to this, the highest honour the College can bestow,

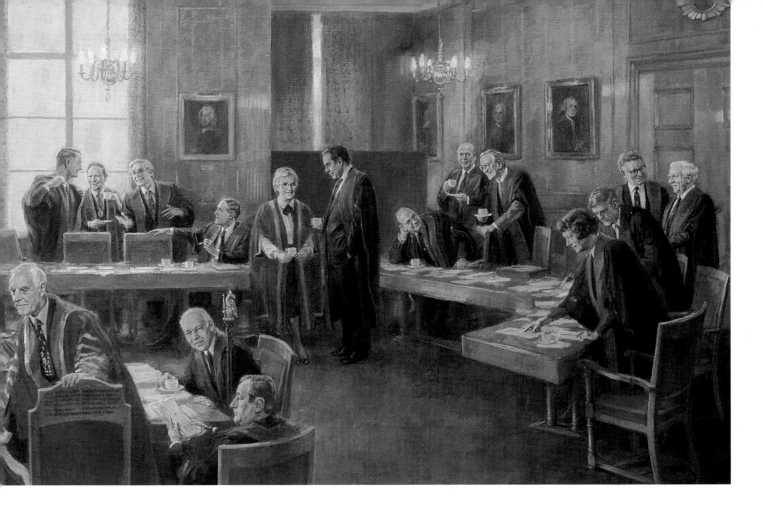

include Sir Winston Churchill and the benefactors Lord Nuffield and Lord Sieff. Medical Honorary Fellows are renowned surgeons and other clinicians from around the world.

The College bestows a large number of medals and lectureships. Many have been amalgamated as the relative value of any financial reward has decreased across two centuries. They include the Hunterian Oration, a lecture delivered biennially by a member of Council; the Hunterian Professorships, awarded in competition for state-of-the-art lectures by experts in their field; and, at the other end of the spectrum, the Preiskel Student Travelling Scholarship, which is awarded to medical students for elective attachments in surgery in the developing world. The Sir Arthur Keith Medal, carrying the portrait of Sir Arthur on one side and the arms of the College on the other, is awarded for distinguished service by members of the College staff or its professional advisers.

In 1956 Council established the Court of Patrons to provide a means of recognising outstanding service to the College. There is no restriction on the size of the Court, and Patrons include past Presidents, distinguished Council members and College benefactors who have retained an active interest in College affairs. The Court meets annually to be updated upon and to discuss College activities.

The Council portrait of 1988 (Fig 6.24), painted at a time of extensive change, features the visionaries who took the College forward into the last decade of the century.

College Publications

For 150 years, the College did not publish a journal, although in 1826 Sir Anthony Carlisle proposed a College publication 'stamped with the authority of the most distinguished men in our profession and authenticated by their names'. The idea floundered when Carlisle failed to obtain the co-operation he needed from the hospitals. Council discussed the possibility of a College publication again in 1930, but the initiative came to nothing. Apart from a single issue of a museum journal in 1892, the matter lay dormant until after the Second World War.

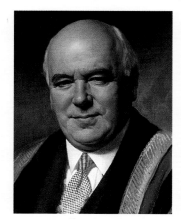

S1 Sir Cecil Pembrey Grey Wakeley (1892-1979)

In 1922, Wakeley joined King's College Hospital, was senior surgeon by 1933 and remained there for the next quarter of a century. He was President of the College from 1949 to 1954, a period that witnessed the completion of the rebuilding of the College, and the establishment of the Faculties of Dental Surgery and Anaesthesia, as well as the academic units and their laboratories. In addition to his work at the *Annals*, he was editor of the *British Journal of Surgery* for 20 years.

By James Gunn

In October 1946 Council established a sub-committee consisting of the President (Sir Alfred Webb-Johnson), the Vice-Presidents (Sir Heneage Ogilvie and Sir Cecil Wakeley) and the Chairman of the Library Committee (Sir Geoffrey Keynes) to consider whether to produce a bulletin to include lecture transcripts and information about forthcoming College activities. At its next meeting, Council approved the committee's recommendation that a journal be published, an editor appointed and an editorial committee established comprising Webb-Johnson, Ogilvie, Wakeley, Keynes, Ernest Finch and Robert McNeill Love. In early 1947, Wakeley became founding editor and chairman of the editorial committee **(Fig S1)**; for the next 22 years, he was indelibly associated with the *Annals*.

The first issue contained a mixture of postgraduate lectures, historical articles, College news, a letter from the President and many advertisements. It included the 1945 Thomas Vicary lecture and review articles covering gangrene and gastric surgery. College news featured short articles on the library during the Second World War as well as one on the pathology museum. This issue set a style and level of quality maintained throughout Wakeley's tenure as editor. A number of College Presidents and other notable names in surgery from the UK and overseas contributed to the journal. The early volumes are goldmines of information on post-war history.

S2 Professor Anthony Harding Rains (b. 1920)

Rains trained at St Mary's Hospital, London, and in Birmingham before becoming Professor of Surgery at Charing Cross Hospital, London. Rains served on Council from 1972 to 1984, was a member of the Court of Examiners 1968-74, was a Hunterian Trustee in 1982 and held the office of Vice-President in 1983. He was Dean of the Institute of Basic Medical Sciences from 1976 to 1982. Rains edited the *Annals* from 1969 to 1983.

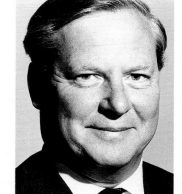

S2

In 1969 Wakeley passed the editorial mantle to Professor Tony Harding Rains, who had been assistant editor for two years **(Fig S2)**. Associate editors in anaesthesia and dental surgery were appointed and the cover was redesigned. Contents remained almost entirely confined to the statutory lectures and postgraduate lectures from College courses. History retained heavy emphasis.

S3 Raymond (Jerry) Kirk (b. 1923)

Trained at the Charing Cross and Royal Free Hospitals, Kirk became a consultant surgeon at the Royal Free Hospital. He was President of the Medical Society of London and of the Surgical Section of the Royal Society of Medicine. Kirk has been the author of numerous surgical texts. He served on Council from 1983 to 1991, was actively involved in the College's Overseas Doctors Training scheme, and was Editor of the *Annals* from 1983 to 1992.

The first radical change in policy came in 1974, when the journal introduced a correspondence section and published short original articles as well as extracts from scientific papers presented at national meetings. These innovations marked the *Annals'* evolution from a house journal to a scientific publication. In the mid-1970s, Council reluctantly decided on financial grounds that the journal should be changed from monthly to bi-monthly.

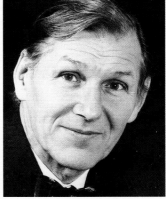

S3

In 1983, in-house news was separated from scientific material with the launch of the *College and Faculty Bulletin* as a loose, eight-page insert within the *Annals*. The following year Jerry Kirk became editor after 12 years as assistant editor (**Fig S3**). Kirk introduced a peer review system through which the *Annals* soon became recognised and accepted for citation by the major bibliographical indexing journals. The *Bulletin* took on a new thrust as a medicopolitical digest.

During this time, the trend in the profession towards sub-specialisation gave rise to a proliferation of journals, while the *Annals* remained focused on the generality of surgery with a powerful clinical base. The new editor in 1992, Barry Jackson, reintroduced carefully selected historical articles. Peer review ensured that quality remained high and, in spite of competition from the specialist journals, a commendable citation index was maintained.

Taking over as editor in 1997, John Lumley was charged by Council to oversee a balanced specialty content with a clinical emphasis: up to one-third of the content of the *Annals* was to consist of peer-reviewed educational articles from invited experts. The *Bulletin* benefited greatly from in-house desktop publishing, its aim being to rapidly report the extensive activities of Council and its Boards, and to invite articles on related topics.

In 1997, Council agreed to the introduction of a Publications Department to reduce printing costs, and to provide an in-house corporate image for the extensive literature covering Board and committee activities. In 1998 the department's proposal to develop a new Internet web site was approved by Council and launched four months later. The site reflected the main activities of the College and provides a key channel to communicate with Fellows, trainees, political decision-makers and members of the public.

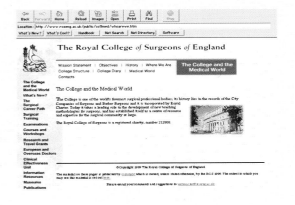

CHAPTER 7

The College Today: The Renaissance *of* the 1990s

7.1 Council of July 1999

(Front row) Peter Leopard, Professor George Bentley, Professor Jack D Hardcastle, John Ll Williams (Vice-President), Barry Jackson (President), Professor Averil Mansfield (Vice-President), Anne Moore, Professor Valerie J Lund. (Second row) Michael Brough, Brian Morgan, Professor Charles Galasko (incoming Vice-President), Michael A Edgar, David J Dandy, Professor Thomas Duckworth, John Carruth, Deirdre Watson. (Third row) Leela Kapila, Professor Peter RF Bell, Ian Barlow, David Rosin, Charles Collins, Hugh Phillips. (Back row) Peter C May, Anthony Catterall, Professor John Fitzpatrick, Professor John SP Lumley, Professor Thomas Treasure, David Barnard, Professor Lewis Spitz, Craig Duncan (Secretary), David J Williams, David Wright.

Members missing from group photograph and pictured below: Linda de Cossart, Professor Bill Heald, Robert HS Lane, Professor Sir Peter Morris, Glenn Neil-Dwyer, Malcolm Pendlebury, Bernard Ribeiro, Christopher Russell.

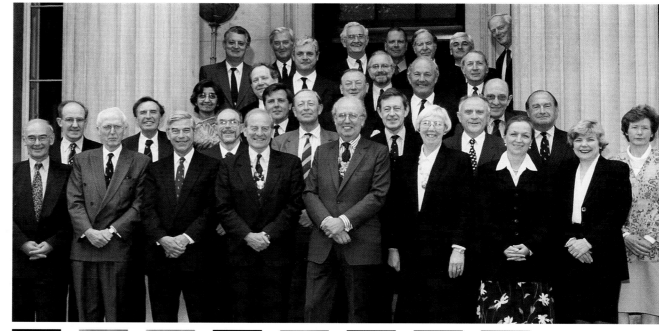

The immediate post-war years were a golden era in College history, with the restoration of its buildings and the blossoming of the Institute of Basic Medical Sciences. However, 30 years on, these research activities had become an unsustainable financial burden that threatened to bleed the College dry. In 1992 Council faced one of the most momentous decisions in its history: whether to support or reject the Hunterian Institute. In the end, Council chose the more controversial option: closure of the Institute.

Over the next decade, Council's decision was vindicated. It achieved a bloodless revolution, and the new direction initiated a renaissance of College activities. The College discovered that donors were happy to support education, and substantial sums were given by Lord Hanson, the Ronald Raven Trust, Lord Wolfson and Mr Danny Hill. The College buildings were redesigned, the development reflecting the changing emphasis from College-based research to education and training. Thus, at its Bicentenary, the College is a vibrant entity, with its Council (Fig 7.1), Fellows and staff addressing current surgical problems and preparing enthusiastically for the challenges of the 21st century.

Renovation of the College Buildings

During the 1960s one major structural problem required attention: the portico had started to lean towards Lincoln's Inn Fields. This was the only part of Charles Dance's 1813 building that Barry had retained, although the west column had been moved to the east to centralise the new, wider building of 1836. Much of Barry's College had been destroyed in the 1941 bombing, but the portico – together with the entrance hall and Library – survived. The portico was prevented from collapsing, but only after hydraulic lifting and underpinning with reinforced concrete.

In the early 1980s, it was a pleasure to walk through Lincoln's Inn Fields, with its magnificent trees and well-kept flowerbeds. By the end of the decade, however, the space had changed to one of litter-strewn lawns and vagrants encroaching onto the College's steps. While the College buildings were dignified, the furnishings and fabric (unchanged for over a quarter of a century) were showing signs of decay. The post-war reconstruction of Barry's building provided a solid outer shell, but its listed exterior was engrained with London's grime.

7.2 Lord Hanson

Lord Hanson is internationally known as an exponent of corporate takeovers. As chairman of Hanson plc (1965–1997), he built a small Yorkshire company into one of the world's largest. He is a founder Trustee of the Hanson Fellowship of Surgery Oxford, a Fellow of the Cancer Research Campaign and an Honorary Fellow of the Royal College of Radiologists.

A number of factors influenced the subsequent changes to the building. First, the Wolfson family contributed £250,000 to provide additional accommodation for the surgical specialist associations. Second, Lord Hanson (Fig 7.2) made a gift to the College of £500,000 to support surgical training other than research, to be expended on building, not staffing. Thus came into being the Hanson Suite of Surgical Training, completed in 1989, which occupies the third and fourth floors within the inner well, above the Hunterian Museum.

Council's ideas further crystallised during 1989, when it was announced that the Queen would open the new Hanson Suite in November. Money from the Frances Gardener Fund was used to clean the external façade, and other funds were found to redecorate the outer, inner and exhibition halls and to replace the railings and gates. The gates had been removed at the beginning of the Second World War;

7.2

7.3 The College today

Photograph by Michael Hurley

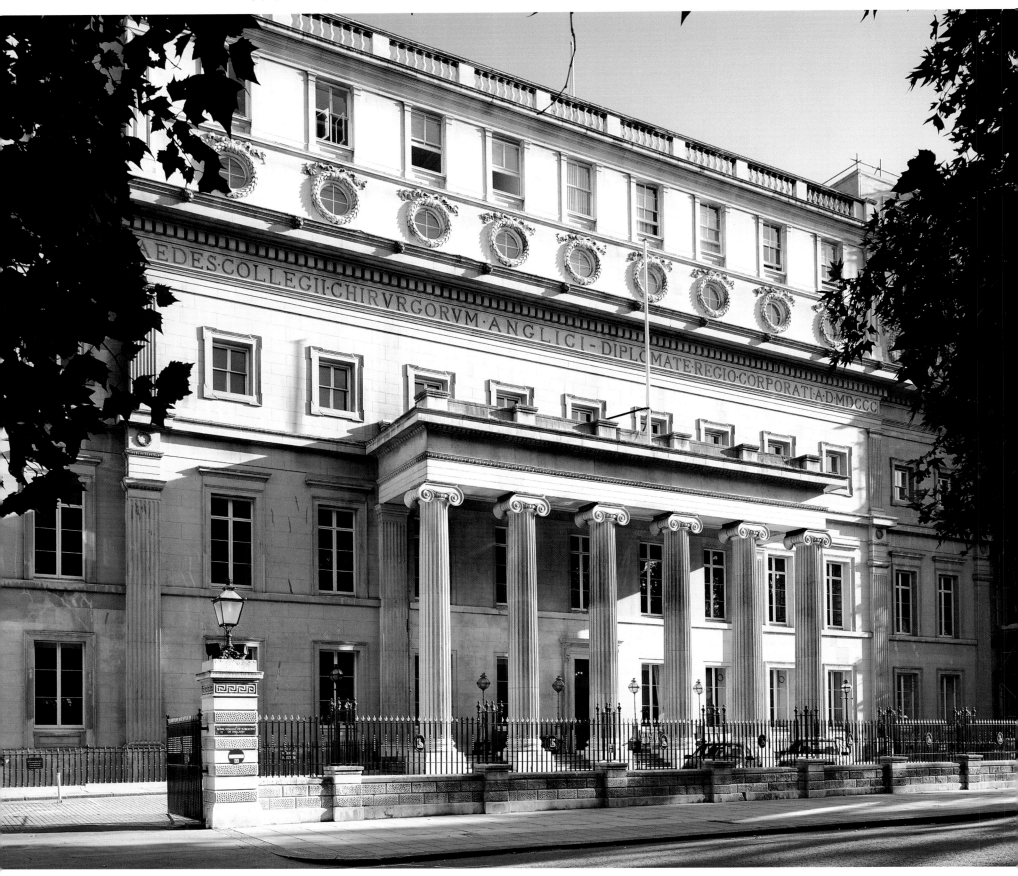

Wilde Sapte, the College solicitors, funded the replacement that restored dignity to the College entrance (Fig 7.3). These donations raised an awareness that charitable monies were available for activities other than research and fuelled Council's resolve to change from a research-centric to an education-based institution.

The closure of the Hunterian Institute between 1992 and 1995 created space within the College at an opportune moment for the proposed educational developments. The rabbit warren of corridors and inaccessible corners were redeveloped, and the laboratory areas that had taken up much floor space were remodelled. Three new lifts were strategically placed to allow rapid access to these areas. The 1950 furnishings, the outdated electrical and heating systems, and the superfluous laboratory gas and plumbing installations were removed and replaced with new cabling and air conditioning. The projected cabling requirements grossly underestimated the subsequent enormous developments in information technology, requiring computers and on-line facilities in every area; further cabling was needed in 1996 and again in 1999.

So it was that the dust and disturbance, which had heralded such a welcome burst of activity in the late 1980s, continued for almost a decade. However, the extensive redevelopment of its facilities – including the establishment of the Ronald Raven Department of Education, the Wolfson Surgical Training Centre, the Blond Training Unit and the Hill Surgical Workshop (see also

7.4 Vandervell Lecture Theatre

Chapter 8) – turned the College into a modern, well-equipped site, ideally suited to the demands of education in the 1990s.

On completion of the education units, Council turned its attention to the ground floor. The No.1 lecture theatre was heavily used and urgently needed refurbishment to bring it up to an acceptable standard for modern audio-visual and telecommunication requirements. The Vandervell trustees agreed that this was an appropriate

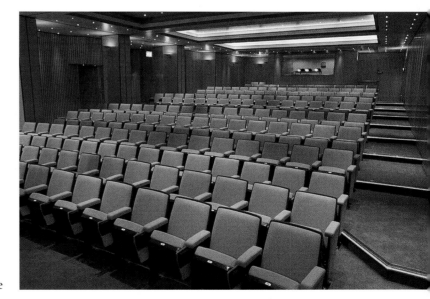

educational development. The upgraded room was renamed the Vandervell Lecture Theatre, and completed in November 1995 at a cost of £750,000 (Fig 7.4).

In July 1997 Council considered plans for new accommodation for the Association of Surgeons of Great Britain and Ireland. Council resolved to fund the building costs of the development across the sixth floor, up to the sum of £200,000, to enable the Association to undertake a £650,000 conversion project. Work started in August 1997 and was completed in April of the following year.

Also in 1997, Council agreed to renovate the entrance and exhibition halls. Experts in Georgian interiors were consulted, and paint scrapings were taken to determine the original colour scheme. They showed nine layers of distemper, paint and varnish in the inner hall, which were a wonderful record of changes in taste over two centuries. The decoration of the inner and outer halls enhanced the staircases and produced a suitable entrance to the Library, the Hunterian Museum and the Raven Department of Education. The result was to regain the Georgian splendour of Barry's building (Fig 7.5).

7.5 The inner College entrance hall as it looks today, with the statue of John Hunter

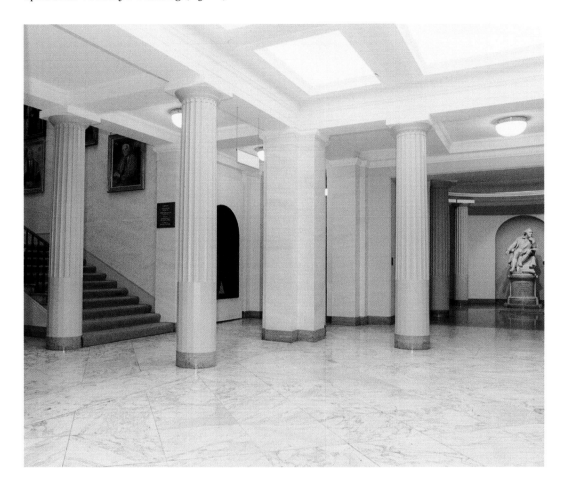

The Nuffield College of Surgical Sciences

The geography of the Nuffield, like that of the College buildings, had not changed significantly through its first quarter century, although regular refurbishments had taken place. Minor modifications did take place to provide the Philip Henman Room, a comfortable sitting room for Fellows and their friends overlooking Lincoln's Inn Fields, and the Howard Gray Room, a large common room.

Council tackled accommodation for its changing clientele. The experiment to upgrade the rooms at the back of the second floor proved to be extremely popular. The plan expanded to upgrade all the bedrooms on the second and third floors, providing en-suite bathrooms or showers with the facilities of a modern hotel. In a sense, the College has become a victim of its own success: the accommodation is in great demand and must be booked well in advance.

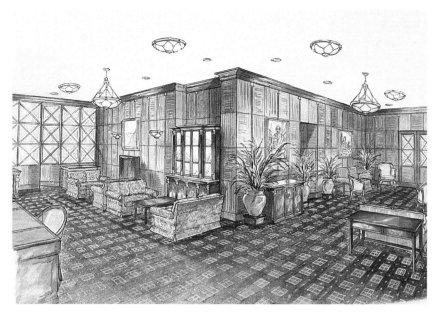
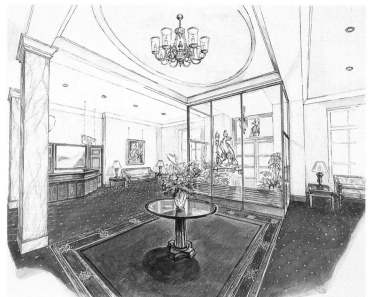

7.6 and 7.7 Designs for remodelling the ground floor of Nuffield College

A bar was opened to complement the Fellows Lounge in the Howard Gray Room, but the location proved to be wrong; it has been relocated in a more appropriate and attractive site, intended to become a focal point for all surgeons working in or visiting London. This Bicentenary Project was planned to convert the whole of the ground floor of the Nuffield, including the area occupied by the Faculty of Dental Surgery, into an elegant common room with a business centre and bar. The project, carried out in late 1999, transformed the derelict lightwell between the new lounge and the Webb-Johnson Hall into a glass-roofed atrium. The design of the area is a sensitive fusion of the modern and traditional (Figs 7.6 and 7.7).

The Properties in Downe

Council resolved in February 1989 that the Buckston Browne Farm should be closed. The College was already leading the trend to reduce the use of animals in research, especially large animals, for which the Buckston Browne Farm had been appropriate. In common with most universities and institutions, the money available for research had become severely constrained, and it was not feasible for the College to continue carrying out research on two sites.

Thus began prolonged discussions on the disposal of the College properties at Downe. In June 1989 a working party considered the future of all these properties. The Trustees of the British Museum (National History) expressed interest in maintaining Down House as a Darwin Museum but believed that it would only be commercially viable if the sandwalk and all the land to the east were included in the estate. The College accepted an offer from the Natural History Museum to provide and pay a member of its staff to act as curator as an interim measure.

In December 1995, after lengthy negotiations, Council resolved that the College should sell Down House and its garden (subject to certain safeguards) and the Buckston Browne Farm to English Heritage: the sale was funded by the Wellcome Trust and completed on 14 February 1996.

The International Office

The College's extensive and distinguished international links (Fig 7.8) can be traced throughout its history. John Hunter frequently had pupils from the United States, and Sir Rickman Godlee (see also Fig 4.15) was present at the inauguration of the American College of Surgeons in 1913.

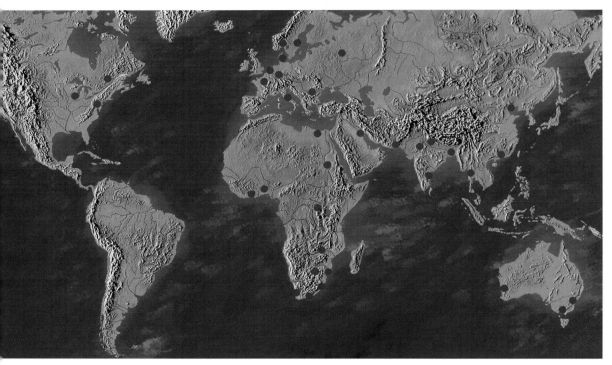

7.8 **Map showing the sites of international office activities**

As overseas health systems and institutions were developed and strengthened, the College benefited from the exchange of ideas with its sister colleges world-wide on how to achieve their shared goal of the highest standards of patient care. The newer colleges, less burdened with history, found innovation easier. They were quicker to change from in-house research to the support of surgical research fellowships, and to introduce exit FRCS examinations.

An example of this international vision was provided by Sir Harry Platt (see also Fig 15.5), who was instrumental in founding the International Federation of Surgical Colleges.

Prominent among the College's activities outside the British Isles has been the holding of the Primary FRCS examination at overseas centres. In addition to conducting the examinations, examiners gave lectures and advice on all manner of problems, and held brainstorming sessions with government ministers and members of the local department of health. Members of the local High Commission or embassy often commented that these fresh and frank thoughts did much for the British image and were greatly appreciated. Examinations often continued when relations between Britain and a particular country were under strain.

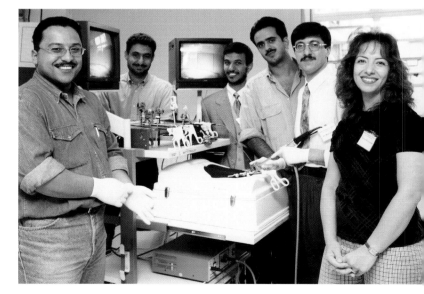

7.9 **Participants from Kuwait on a** *Basic Surgical Skills* **course, October 1997**

7.9

Throughout the College's history, overseas graduates have come to the United Kingdom for further training (Fig 7.9), but frequently had difficulty in obtaining suitable posts in the National Health Service (NHS). No system existed to match candidates with suitable training posts or to provide them with a certificate to mark the successful completion of a specified period of training. For this, the Overseas Doctors Training scheme was developed in the early 1980s (see also Chapter 9).

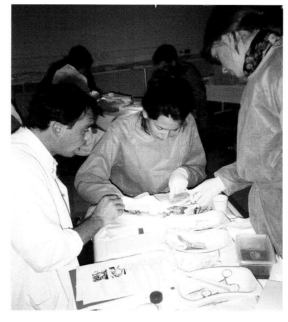

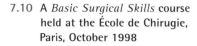

7.10 A *Basic Surgical Skills* course held at the École de Chirugie, Paris, October 1998

In November 1996 the College established an International Office, under the direction of Professor Jack Hardcastle (see also Fig 8.2), to promote the College internationally and to co-ordinate the College's growing international activities. The experience and skill developed in the Raven Department of Education established it as an international resource centre, and it now provides ministries and overseas institutions, both public and private, with educational packages tailored to their local needs. These 'packages' comprise educational programmes ranging from practical skills courses to distance learning projects, advice on development and the delivery of a local curriculum, and help with designing and equipping centres for teaching appropriate skills (Fig 7.10).

In the first year of operation, the International Office received visits and enquiries from over 40 countries. Training programmes were set up in many parts of the world, and international linkages provided two-way communication and allowed expertise to be shared by visits and satellite links. Overseas links have been further fostered by triennial Council visits and joint meetings with fellow surgical colleges. The first was in October 1989, when the College, with the College of Anaesthetists and the Faculty of Dental Surgery, held a joint meeting in Bangkok with the Royal College of Surgeons of Thailand, before moving on to Kuala Lumpur to take part in the 23rd Malaysia Singapore Congress of Medicine. Similar joint meetings have been held in Karachi and Delhi, Abu Dhabi and Colombo, and more recently in Harare and Cape Town (Fig 7.11).

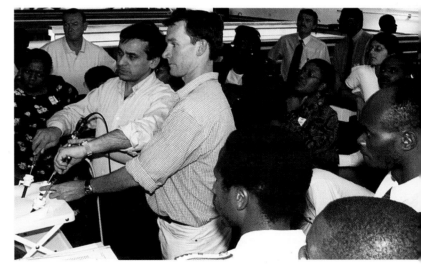

7.11 Professor Ara Darzi demonstrating laparoscopic techniques at a surgical training workshop in Harare, Zimbabwe, 1998

7.11

Clinical Governance

As the 20th century drew to its close and the NHS approached its 50th Anniversary, the new Labour government presented its health policy. This had profound implications for every hospital and healthcare professional by introducing the concept of clinical governance, making it the statutory duty of every health organisation both to maintain standards and to improve the quality of care.

At the same time, the General Medical Council (GMC) found itself dealing with the alleged poor clinical performance of three doctors involved with children's cardiac surgery at the Bristol Royal Infirmary (Fig 7.12). The issue was later subject to a public inquiry at which evidence was taken from all related governing medical bodies as well as the College President.

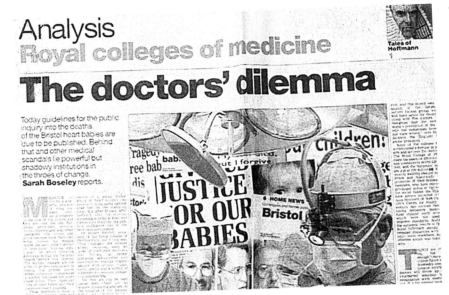

7.12

Reprinted with permission of *The Guardian*

Through the period 1984 to 1995, for which the Bristol Royal Infirmary inquiry was taking evidence, the College had no formal statutory power to control the quality of those appointed to consultant posts. The European Specialist Medical Qualifications Order in 1995 made it mandatory (from January 1997) for a candidate for a consultant appointment to be entered on the new Specialist Register of the GMC. Through this legislation the College now has the ability to regulate entry to the consultant grade.

The College is also collaborating with the GMC in putting in place a system of revalidation to remain on the medical Register, and to ensure that fully trained and experienced surgeons keep up to date throughout their careers. The College has developed a 'rapid response' mechanism to enable independent investigation of alleged unsatisfactory surgical practice in any hospital. A Patient Liaison Group has been established to promote greater openness and understanding.

Surgery is particularly vulnerable to criticism. Operative procedures can be difficult, and the outcome cannot be guaranteed. Complications may be disabling or lethal. It is essential that evidence-based markers are obtained with which to identify poor performance and to intervene before any clinical hazard arises. The College has been particularly active through its Clinical Effectiveness Unit in working with the specialty associations to identify appropriate marker procedures in each surgical field.

The recently established Professional Standards Committee advises Council on all matters related to quality of surgical practice, clinical governance, rapid response and pastoral care. It also has the responsibility for effective collaboration with internal and external bodies on all matters related to the quality of clinical practice.

College Governance Today

The main work of Council is currently carried out by six Boards (Education, Training, Examinations, Research, External Affairs and Finance) and a series of committees reporting directly to Council. Each Board is served by a Secretary and a team of College staff (Fig 7.13). Council members may serve on up to three Boards, as can invited members, regional advisers, tutors, educational tutors, specialty representatives and other surgical experts (Figs 7.14 and 7.15).

7.13 Secretary Roger Duffett and team

From left to right: David Munn, Craig Duncan, Maria Coonick, Roger Duffett, Helen Allgrove, Martyn Coomer and Peter Roberts, 1997.

Council remains sensitive to the distribution of specialists within its ranks. In 1988 co-opted members were invited from neurology, paediatrics and plastic surgery. In 1989 the co-opted member system, which had been in effect since 1947, was replaced by one whereby representatives were invited from the nine specialist associations with a specialist advisory committee, and from accident and emergency medicine. Additional representatives came from the Court of Examiners, Surgeons in Training and sister colleges, including the newly formed Royal College of Ophthalmologists. Reciprocal representation of sister colleges ceased in 1995.

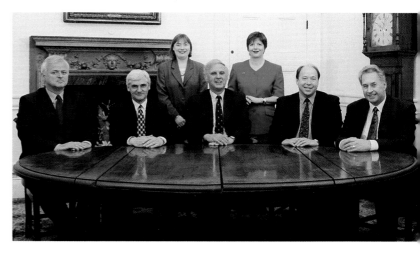

7.14 Recent Presidents of the College

From left to right: Sir Norman Browse, Sir Geoffrey Slaney, Lord Smith, Sir Rodney Sweetnam, Sir Reginald Murley, Sir Ian Todd, Sir Terence English.

The Faculty of Anaesthetists (see also Chapter 12) became an independent College of Anaesthetists in October 1988 but remained within the College buildings until 1992. At that time it was also granted its own Royal Charter.

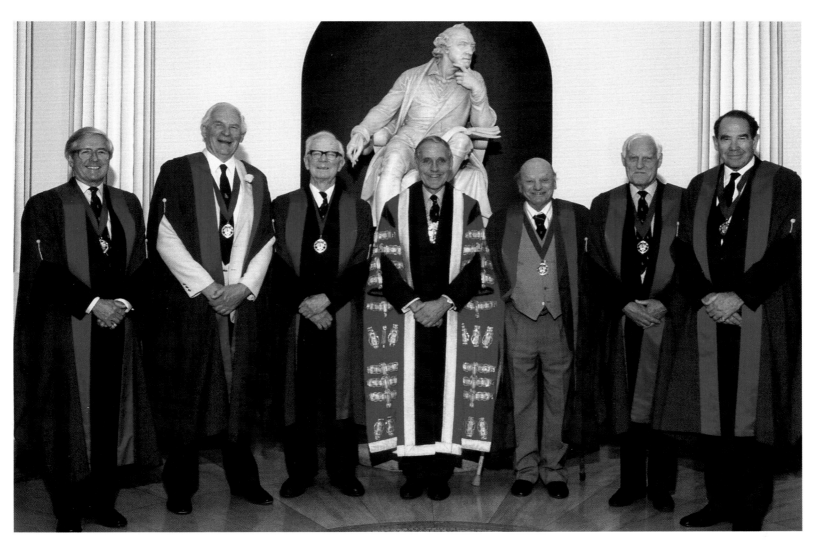

7.15 Council of 1997

From left to right: Anne Moore, Peter Leopard, Charles Collins, Professor John Lumley, Professor Valerie Lund, David Dandy, John Carruth, Professor Peter Bell, Professor Charles Galasko, Brian Morgan, Professor Averil Mansfield, Brendan Devlin, Roger Duffett (Secretary), Professor Jack Hardcastle (Vice-President), Sir Rodney Sweetnam (President), Professor Bill Heald (Vice-President), Professor Thomas Duckworth, Professor Sir Peter Morris, Barry Jackson, Professor George Bentley, Leela Kapila, Peter May, Craig Duncan (proleptic Secretary), David Rosin, John Ll Williams, Michael Edgar, Hugh Phillips, Professor Thomas Treasure, John Williams.

By Boyd & Evans

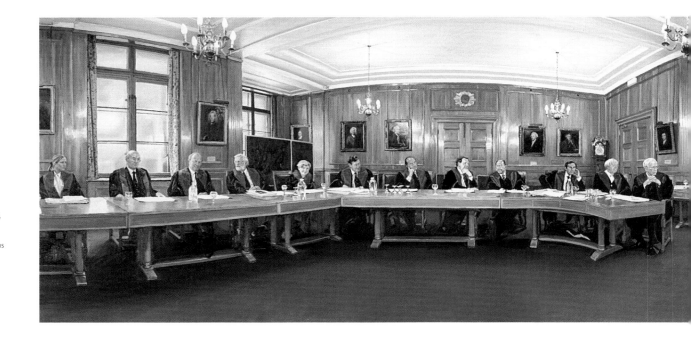

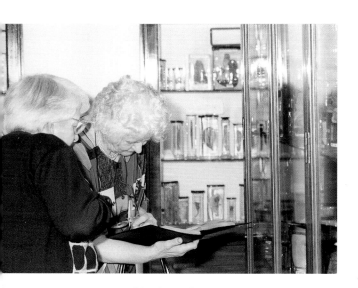

7.16 Members of the public visiting the Museum during Open Day, 1998

In July 1999 an additional invited Council member was introduced from the Welsh Board. The Board had been formed in 1989 and had itself developed from the Standing Committee for Wales, founded in 1985. Previous representation from the Board had been by a Council member who was living in Wales, but this arrangement had not necessarily guaranteed representation.

The debate over how to equate the privileges and status of elected and invited Council members continues. The problem relates to the term of office: the tenure of specialist representatives, usually three years, is similar to membership of the parent Council and ensures that invited members are abreast of current matters within their specialty. Elected members, however, represent the generality of surgery for a term of ten years (six plus four, from 1997), which gives them time to learn how the College works and to direct its activities.

The first woman to be elected to Council was Phyllis George, in 1979. She subsequently became Vice-President in 1988. At the millennium, the number of women Council members had increased to five. The first Faculty of Anaesthetists Council member to become Vice-President was Professor Sir Gordon Robson (see also Fig 12.14), in 1977, and in 1992, John Rayne was the first Council member from the Faculty of Dental Surgery to hold this office.

Membership

Fellows and Members of another College, and those with equivalent training from overseas, can be sponsored by a Fellow for *ad eundem* Fellowship or Membership. The annual Fellowship subscription introduced in 1957 was initially five guineas, but progressively increased. The full Fellowship subscription at the millennium is £250 for UK resident surgeons; this fee is reduced for surgeons from other countries, for surgeons within six years of passing the examination, and for those who are retired. The current College membership figures are 14,000 FRCS and

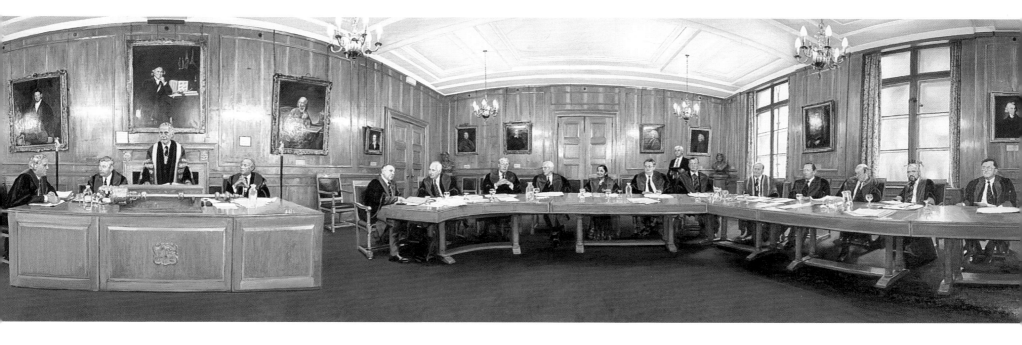

2,400 FDS. There are also 3,000 Affiliate Members who are surgeons-in-training, usually studying on the College distance learning course. The latter are not charged a subscription but receive a range of information and publications, including the College *Bulletin*.

Road Shows

For several years the College has undertaken regular road shows, where the President, members of Council and the Court of Examiners, other senior surgeons and members of staff visit local centres and meet surgeons of all levels. Speakers outline current issues and initiatives in their field, and this is followed by discussion of these specific and general topics. The President and Council greatly value these meetings for the feedback on a range of College policies and activities, and for insight gained into local issues and problems.

Another aspect of the College's ongoing activities around the country is a series of career days organised for medical students and pre-registration and senior house officers. These events promote surgery as a career and outline opportunities in the various specialties. Students and trainees are encouraged to affiliate with the College at the earliest opportunity to take advantage of the many benefits it offers professionally and socially. Open days for the public include lectures and guided tours of the College; the museums can be visited by arrangement (Fig 7.16).

The College's first regional office was opened in Newcastle-upon-Tyne in December 1997 (Fig 7.17). Housed in the postgraduate centre at the Freeman Hospital, by kind agreement of the clinical tutor and postgraduate dean, this is a joint venture with the Royal College of Physicians of London. Its success has stimulated the extension of the programme, and a Welsh office was established in Cardiff in November 1999.

7.17 Opening of the Northern Office, 1997

From left to right: Professor Sir George Alberti, President of the Royal College of Physicians of London, George Proud, Regional Adviser for the Northern Region, Lorraine Waugh, Northern Office Administrator, and Sir Rodney Sweetnam, then President of the College.

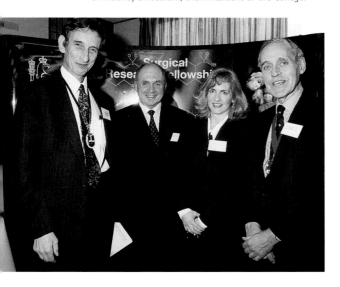

The Senate

In the late 1980s, there was a desire among the specialist associations to discuss matters of mutual interest, in particular higher surgical training and the development of specialist Fellowship examinations. This resulted in the foundation of the Federation of Surgical Specialist Associations. In 1993, at one of the Joint Meetings of Surgical Colleges, it was decided to reconstitute the body as The Senate of the Royal Surgical Colleges of Great Britain and Ireland and to invite the President or another representative of each of the nine surgical specialist associations and the Faculty of Accident and Emergency Medicine to join them. The first meeting of the Senate was held in September 1993. The Joint Committee for Higher Surgical Training and the Joint Committee on Intercollegiate Examinations became sub-committees of the Senate.

Two years later, the name of the group was changed to The Senate of Surgery of Great Britain and Ireland, and the chairmen of the Joint Committee on Continuing Medical Education and the Joint Committee on European Affairs became members. The Senate meets quarterly.

Social Activities

The social aspect of College life is an integral part of its existence. Each Diplomates Day is an open day, when new Diplomates, their relatives and friends explore the historic collections,

7.18 Diplomates Day procession

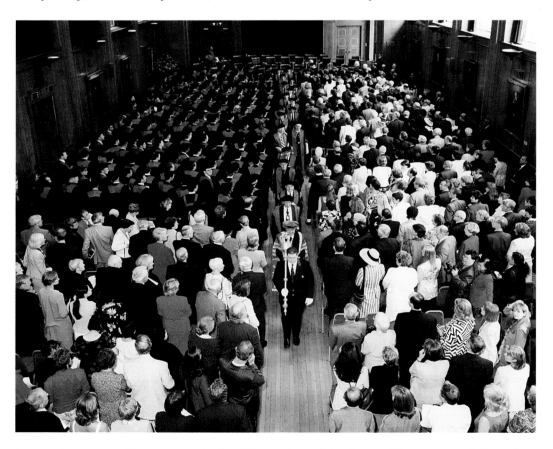

browse through the Library, and mingle with members of the Court of Examiners and Council (Fig 7.18). The day ends with a dinner in the Edward Lumley Hall.

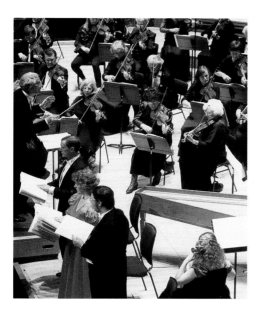

7.19 The gala performance of Anne Hunter's translation of *The Creation* with the Hunterian Festival Choir and Orchestra

7.20 Anne Hunter's manuscript

Anne Hunter, John's wife, supplied Franz Joseph Haydn with words for two very successful sets of English canzonettas in 1794 and 1795. On hearing the first performance of Haydn's *The Creation* in London in 1800, Anne Hunter was unhappy with the English translation of the words, drawn from Genesis and Milton's *Paradise Lost*. Perhaps it was the letter from a friend commenting on how 'lamentable to see such divine music joined with such miserable, broken English' that motivated Anne to write another version. It is not known whether the old Master ever saw Anne Hunter's libretto, but the manuscript was donated to the College, together with some of John Hunter's papers, in 1926. Lord Smith's reference to the manuscript in his Hunterian Oration of 1977 was noted by Council member Aileen Adams, a singer who had a particular interest in medical history. Haydn scholar HC Robbins Landon proclaimed it a fascinating discovery and worthy of publication.

7.21 The College's float in the 1996 Lord Mayor's Procession passing St Paul's Cathedral

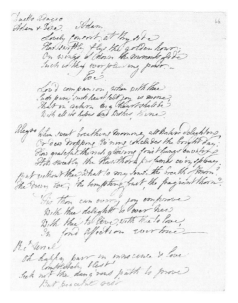

7.20

The Council cricket and golf teams are of mixed talent. Not all can emulate the county cricketing experience of the late Lord Smith, or the enthusiasm of John Carruth, its Secretary. The match with the College staff has many features of a clan war, and has provided many memorable moments.

An historic event occurred in 1993: the bicentenary of the death of John Hunter coincided with the College's hosting the third European Congress of Surgery in London. The Hunter Festival Chorus and Orchestra, conducted by John Lumley, gave the first performance of Anne Hunter's translation of Haydn's *The Creation* in the Royal Festival Hall in September under the patronage of HC Robbins Landon (Figs 7.19 and 7.20). The support of Glaxo Holdings plc enabled an Anne Hunter Research Fellowship to be funded out of the proceeds of the concert.

In 1996 John Chalstrey, a Fellow of the College, became the first surgeon to be Lord Mayor of London. Council celebrated the occasion, together with the Company of Barbers, by jointly manning a float in the Lord Mayor's Procession around the City of London (Fig 7.21).

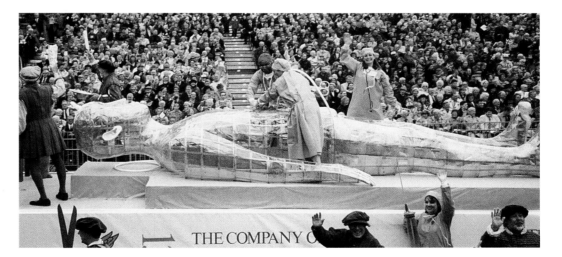

A Senior Fellows Society was founded in 1999 with Adrian Marston, past Vice-President, as its first chairman. All Fellows of the College who have reached retirement are eligible. Activities are social rather than professional, except for assisting in the work of the College when required.

Council appointed Professor Valerie Lund, Council member, to oversee the College Bicentenary celebrations: they include a ball, a banquet, a gala of music and verse covering the last two centuries, and a national service of thanksgiving at St Paul's Cathedral. Surgeon artists were invited to pull out their old masterpieces or prepare new ones for an art exhibition: the *Bulletin* previewed the event by using a series of surgeons' paintings for its cover illustrations.

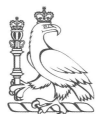

The Raven Department *of* Education: A Centre *of* Excellence for Surgical Teaching

Council decided in 1992 to make the College a centre of excellence for teaching surgeons at all stages of their training and professional lives. Inspired by the President, Sir Norman Browse (Fig 8.1), the College recognised that the limited range of courses available during the days of the Hunterian Institute needed to be extended into carefully tailored and comprehensive teaching programmes. To realise its educational vision, the College needed to provide a highly

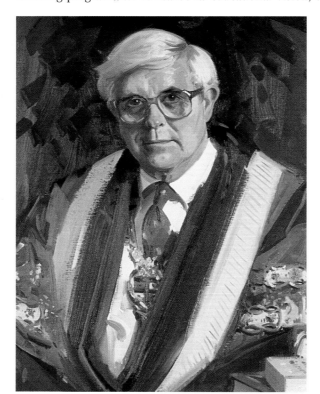

8.1 Professor Sir Norman Leslie Browse (b. 1931)

Norman Browse was elected to Council in 1986 and President 1992–95. This period saw the establishment of the Raven Department of Education, together with the Wolfson Basic Surgical Skills Centre and the Danny Hill Advanced Skills Surgical Centre, the Lumley Study Centre and the refurbishment of the Nuffield College. He was Reader in Surgery, Professor of Vascular Surgery, Professor of Surgery and Head of Department at St Thomas's Hospital between 1965 and 1996.

By Andrew Festing

specialised environment in which trainees and consultants could study surgery and acquire and practise surgical skills in a safe and structured way. Aware that it is not always appropriate or practical for surgeons to attend courses in central London, Council made it a central theme for its proposed education department to conceive courses that could be taken in other parts of the country.

Strong leadership was needed to take the College's educational ambitions forward: Jack Hardcastle was appointed as Director of Education, and early in 1993 Helen Allgrove joined the College as Education Secretary (Fig 8.2). In addition to the small number of academic and administrative staff who were already involved in College courses,

8.2 Professor Jack Hardcastle and Helen Allgrove

Jack Hardcastle was appointed Senior Lecturer in the Department of Surgery at The London Hospital in 1968 and Foundation Professor of Surgery in The University of Nottingham and Honorary Consultant to the Nottingham Hospitals in 1970. Hardcastle has been President of the Surgical Research Society, The British Association of Surgical Oncology, and the Sections of Surgery and Coloproctology at The Royal Society of Medicine. He was elected to Council in 1987, and became Vice-President in 1995. He was appointed Director of Education in 1992 and Director of International Activities in 1997.

Helen Allgrove was appointed as Secretary to the Education Board in 1993 and in that capacity was in administrative charge of the Education Department. She was a driving force and leader of a team of professional educators responsible for the development of a comprehensive programme of surgical education from trainees through to consultant level.

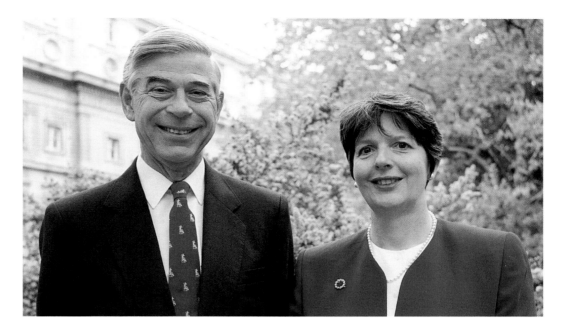

the department gradually built up highly effective multi-disciplinary teams that included (in addition to visiting surgeons) basic scientists, educators and technical support staff. The department appointed a number of part-time educational tutors to guide many of its projects. Without their help and dedication the department could not have grown in the way it has.

Creating a Teaching Environment

Following the closure of several research departments in Lincoln's Inn Fields, the College reassigned the whole fourth floor of the building and a generous portion of the first floor to the new department. Between 1992 and 1995, a succession of major capital projects gradually transformed these areas from scientific laboratories into a suite of state-of-the-art teaching facilities, a modern study centre and an administrative base. In addition to the College's investment of its own resources, a number of significant donations and grants from outside the College helped greatly to develop the department's facilities and individual courses.

8.3 Ronald William Raven (1904–1991)

From his early days as a prize-winning student at St Bartholomew's Hospital to his establishment of the Ronald Raven Department of Clinical Oncology at the Royal Free Hospital and the Ronald Raven Chair of Clinical Oncology, Raven's career was marked by enormous contributions to the treatment of cancer. He was Master of the Worshipful Company of Barbers, founder of several oncological associations, and author of books on both medical and theological topics. He served as Chairman and then President of the charitable Marie Cure Foundation. Raven's association with the College spanned some 60 years, during which time he was an active fundraiser, Hunterian Professor, Erasmus Wilson Demonstrator, Arris and Gale Lecturer, and member of Council.

By WJ Rowden

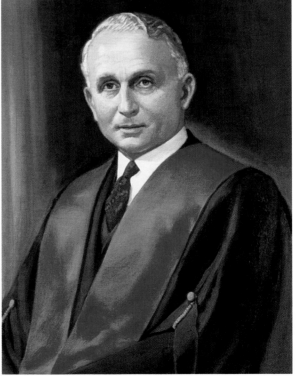

8.3

The Raven Department of Education was named after Ronald Raven (Fig 8.3), a former member of Council whose courses were emulated by many. His passion for surgical education was combined with a conviction that the College should take a strong lead

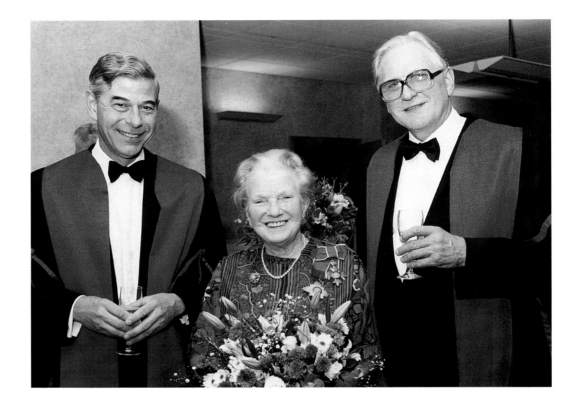

8.4 Dame Kathleen Raven opening the Raven Department of Education

An important member of the medical profession herself, Dame Kathleen (1910–1999) was the Chief Nursing Officer of the United Kingdom from 1958 to 1972. She is shown here with Jack Hardcastle and Alan Lettin, Vice-President.

in providing that education. A generous bequest from the trustees of Raven's estate, made possible by his sister Dame Kathleen Raven, enabled the completion of the first floor reception area and offices; these changes brought together for the first time most of the key surgeons and permanent staff involved in setting up the department. Dame Kathleen officially opened the department in September 1993 (Fig 8.4).

8.5 Council member David Dandy instructing on an orthopaedic workshop in knee replacement

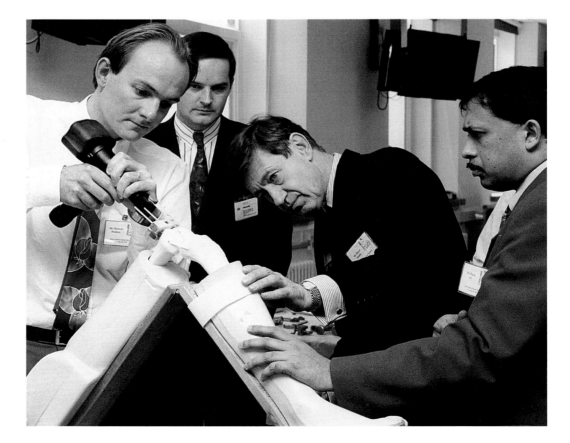

Wolfson Surgical Training Centre

Until 1992, any courses at the College that involve practical teaching had to be held on the ground floor. The Edward Lumley Hall had to be temporarily converted into workshops (Fig 8.5). Reconstruction of the fourth floor changed all this, beginning with the Wolfson Surgical Training Centre, a splendid set of multi-purpose workshops funded by the Wolfson Foundation (Fig 8.6).

Blond Training Unit

In the early 1990s, a new surgical technology – keyhole or minimal access surgery – burst onto the scene. Following several widely reported incidents, the public questioned whether the surgical profession was prepared to use this technique and began to ask, 'Is my surgeon competent to do my operation?' Lord Wolfson responded by offering £1.5 million to help the teaching of minimal access surgery. This figure was matched by a similar sum from the government, and bids were invited from across the country.

8.6

8.6 Lord Wolfson (b. 1927)

Leonard Gordon Wolfson, Founder Trustee of the Wolfson Foundation since 1955, has served as Chairman of Great Universal Stores since 1981 and Burberrys Ltd since 1978. A long-standing patron of the College, Wolfson received an honorary FRCS in 1988.

The College was chosen as one of three national training centres for teaching the new surgical techniques. To equip itself to fulfil this role, the College refurbished the fourth floor and converted it within a year into a unique facility for teaching the practical skills of minimal access surgery in several medical disciplines. When Gerald Malone, Minister of Health, formally opened the new facility in February 1995, he saw trainees using the teaching laboratory, its specially commissioned simulators and a demonstration of the state-of-the-art video links to the College's original clinical partners in the project, The Royal London Hospital and the Royal Surrey County Hospital. In 1999 a substantial donation from the Neville and Elaine Blond Charitable Trust enabled the College to keep up with the rapidly changing technology; this part of the Wolfson Surgical Training Centre was named the Blond Training Unit.

The Blond Training Unit is equipped with state-of-the-art workstations, specially designed to the College's specification. High-quality equipment and instrumentation suitable for each of the nine SAC-recognised surgical specialties is complemented by a range of simulators suitable for teaching a graded sequence of videoendoscpoic exercises. Practical skills training sessions are supplemented by lectures, group discussions and live television transmissions of operative procedures.

8.7 Hill Surgical Workshop

The Hill Surgical Workshop simulates the operating conditions of a modern hospital and boasts a high standard of equipment for all specialties of surgery. A controlled, air-conditioned environment allows for all aspects of anatomical teaching, supported by services including irrigation, suction and compressed air. Audio-visual facilities relay a tutor's demonstration to monitors around the room, so that participants can view all demonstrations clearly from their workstations as well as observe operations via live links into operating theatres.

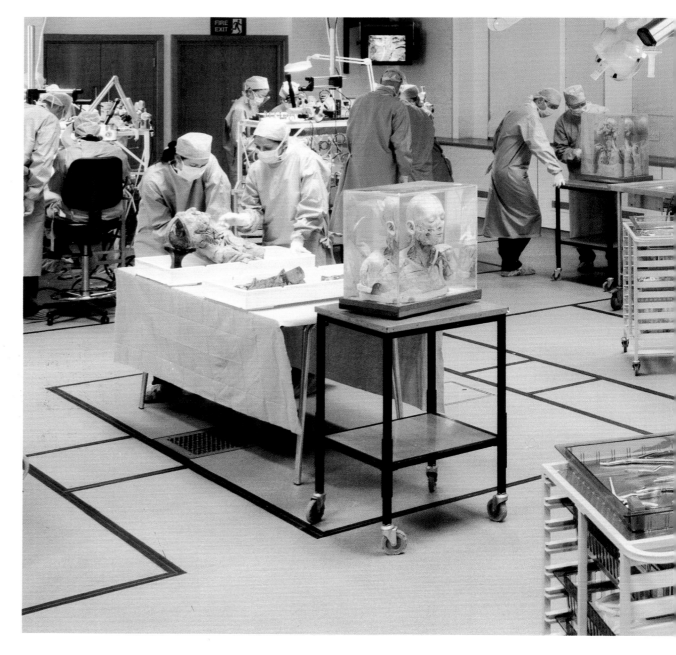

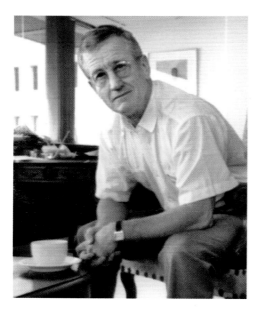

8.8 Danny Hill (b. 1942)

Born in Belfast, Northern Ireland, Danny Hill moved to Australia after school. He developed a taste for the stock market and went on to build a fortune in property and investment. After undergoing surgery in London, Hill became convinced of the importance of teaching surgeons using a hands-on approach. He takes a personal interest in the running of the Hill Surgical Workshop and in the establishment of a sister unit to be opened in Perth, Western Australia, in May 2000.

8.9 The audio-visual control room co-ordinates the College's interactive surgical telecommuncations network

Hill Surgical Workshop

The surgical skills teaching facility culminated in May 1996 with the Hill Surgical Workshop (Fig 8.7), following a generous donation by Danny Hill (Fig 8.8). The workshop uses cadaver material and surgical prosection in teaching advanced surgical skills to consultants and advanced trainees. This provides the ideal facility for teaching anatomy, which is still vital for the trainee surgeon. It is the setting for masterclasses for the experienced surgeon and is the only such facility in Europe. To achieve its full potential, the Hill Surgical Workshop required a sophisticated audio-visual infrastructure to allow operating

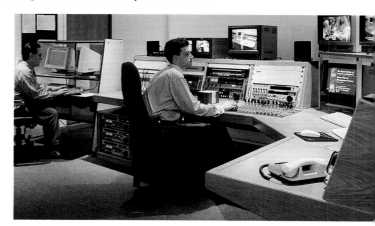

8.9

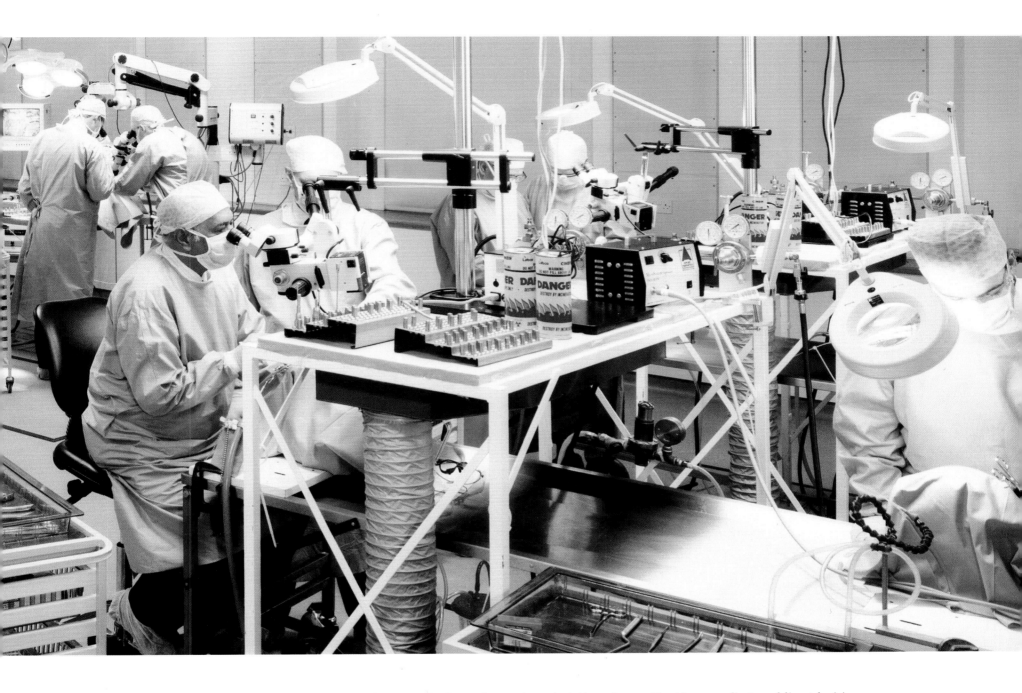

microscopes to be used at each work station, along with video recordings and live television pictures from clinical centres (Fig 8.9). The funding for this component of the project was donated by the Worshipful Company of Barbers, from whose generosity the Raven Department of Education has benefited in many other ways since its inception.

Lumley Study Centre

On the first floor of the Library, the Coulthurst Room was used to centralise all journals and books published in the previous ten years. Thanks to the financial support of two far-sighted members of the College Court of Patrons, Richard and Henry Lumley, the Lumley Study Centre was opened in December 1994 (see also Chapter 16). As well as specialist literature, it encompasses computers and video machines so that, for the first time, surgeons can pursue their studies at the College in a truly multimedia centre.

The Scope of Courses

The College is concerned with the education of surgeons throughout their entire careers. The Raven Department of Education was established at a time when changes taking place in the health service highlighted the need for changes in postgraduate surgical education. Surgical training was shortened to bring the UK into line with the rest of Europe. Following a report in 1993 by the then Chief Medical Officer, Sir Kenneth Calman (see also Fig 10.4), training was divided into two stages: basic principles of surgery in general followed by training in a chosen surgical specialty. It is now possible, at least in theory, for a surgeon to complete training within seven years of qualification: a period similar to that in North America and the rest of Europe.

During the first five years of the Raven Department of Education, a comprehensive programme of courses was developed to cover the new curriculum for senior house officers (SHOs) preparing for the new MRCS. More advanced specialised courses were planned in conjunction with many of the specialist associations aimed at the specialist registrars who were working towards the Intercollegiate FRCS. Masterclasses for consultants were introduced and immediately proved popular.

Senior House Officers

The College has responsibility for the training and assessment of trainees during their basic surgical training period. SHOs could not always be expected to travel to the College, so wherever possible, courses were offered near their place of work. The range of learning opportunities now available to SHOs at regional centres shows how far the Raven Department of Education has developed alternatives to courses based in London.

8.10 Bill Thomas, Blond Surgical Skills Tutor, teaching on the *Basic Surgical Skills* course

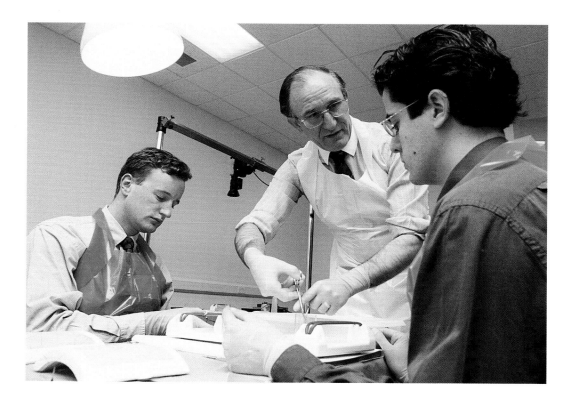

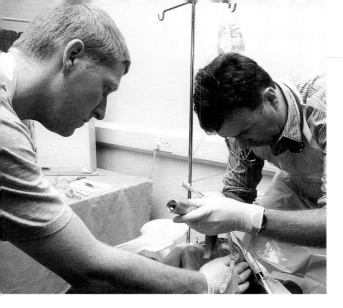

8.11 Practising airway and ventilation techniques on an *Advanced Trauma Life Support* course for instructors

At the beginning of their careers, SHOs must be taught principles of safe practice and simple practical skills, such as knot-tying and suturing, that will last throughout their professional lives. The *Basic Surgical Skills* course was developed and became an intercollegiate activity, with the four surgical Colleges agreeing upon a syllabus. The Royal College of Surgeons of England then led the development of the course and the production of course materials. This course is now a mandatory part of training and is held in 49 centres throughout England and Wales. It is completed by some 1,100 trainees each year (Fig 8.10).

Two other courses highly recommended for basic surgical trainees are also run at regional centres in England and Wales. In the American College of Surgeon's course *Advanced Trauma Life Support*, trainees learn the skills necessary to treat injured patients (Fig 8.11) using simulated patients, as does the *Care of the Critically Ill Surgical Patient* course, which teaches how to manage critically ill surgical patients on the ward (Fig 8.12).

8.12 Simulated patient assessment on a *Care of the Critically Ill Surgical Patient* course

In addition to developing surgical skills through clinical training and carefully structured courses, SHOs must study surgical science and the applied basic sciences relevant to their profession. Work had begun under the Hunterian Institute on a distance learning course: the Surgeons in Training Education Programme (*STEP*). The *STEP* course covers the knowledge needed for the MRCS diploma and complements the short practical courses as well as everyday experience in the operating theatre or at the bedside. Launched in August 1996 and now in its second edition, *STEP* comprises ten modules with associated readers and audio tapes.

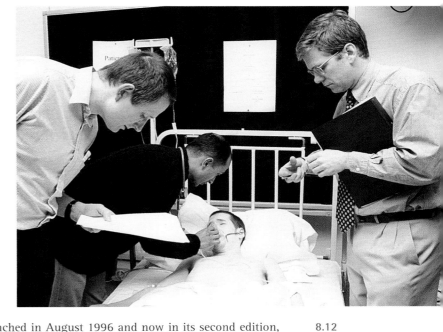

8.12

STEP has proved highly popular with trainees and their consultant trainers, many of whom now plan local teaching programmes that support and extend the *STEP* modules. Trainees are brought together two or three times a year, filling the College with enthusiastic young surgeons. In its first few years, over 2,000 trainees enrolled in *STEP*. The efficacy of *STEP* is shown by the pass rate of its members.

Through these educational programmes for young surgeons, the Raven Department of Education has involved the College with every trainees, including those whose work makes it difficult to come to London to study.

Specialist Registrars

As trainees enter higher surgical training in their chosen specialties, the Raven Department of Education provides highly focused courses to assist in their professional development. These advanced skills courses for senior trainees and consultants have been developed in partnership with the specialist associations (Figs 8.13 and 8.14).

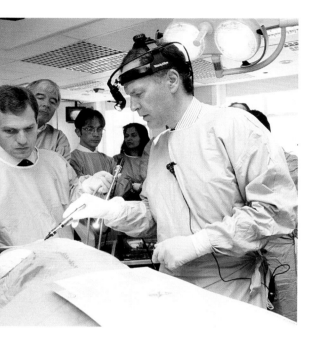

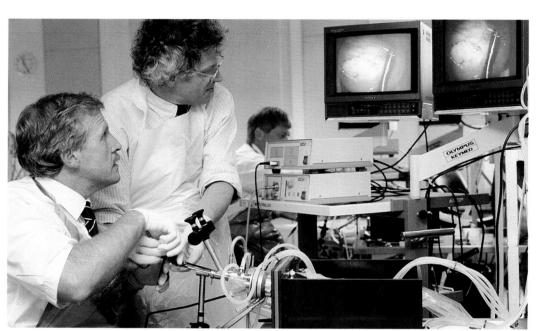

8.14

8.13 Andrew Baildam with Marcus Galea on the *Fundamental Techniques in Breast Reconstruction* course

8.14 Professor Gerhard Buess from Germany teaching on the *Transanal Endoscopic Microsurgery* course

Advanced skills courses utilise the television links to specialised hospitals, which were first introduced for the Minimal Access Therapy Training Unit and the Hill Surgical Workshop. Today live operations in many different hospitals can be viewed in skills teaching laboratories. Participants may pose questions to the operating surgeon and discuss issues and techniques through the course director, who acts as moderator. This network enables surgeons with a particular expertise to play an important practical part in teaching for the College from their own operating theatres.

Consultants

The Raven Department of Education has developed a wide-ranging programme of continuing medical education and professional development to help consultant surgeons keep their skills and knowledge up to date.

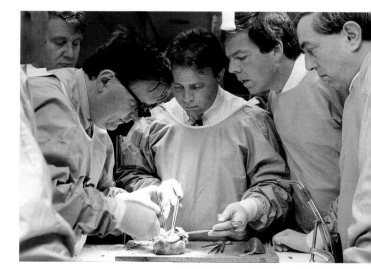

8.15 John Pepper instructing a group of consultants on the advanced course, *Aortic Root Surgery: Homograft, Autograft and Stentless Porcine Valve*

Based at first on the Hill Surgical Workshop, surgical masterclasses now give consultants an opportunity to work with international experts and learn the latest techniques in an environment that simulates the operating theatre (Fig 8.15). As well as specialised skills courses, consultants follow courses of more general interest, such as medicolegal issues and medical management.

8.15

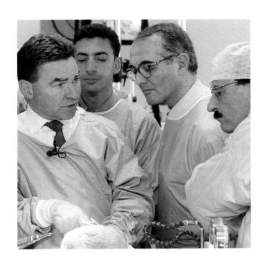

8.16 Alan Crockard instructing on the anatomical masterclass *Transoral Approaches to the Skull Base*

This class has been transmitted in a live, three-way audio-visual link from the Chinese University in Hong Kong to Australia and Singapore.

Assuring the Quality of Courses

In developing and piloting new courses, the Raven Department of Education pays attention to monitoring the quality of teaching and learning. A key plank in the quality assurance of College courses was the introduction of *Training the Trainers* courses, to train the teaching faculty for the courses and improve the teaching skills of consultants throughout the country. Since the first course, some 1,000 consultants have benefited.

Continuing Medical Education

In 1995 the Senate agreed to introduce a scheme to record consultants' participation in continuing medical education and continued professional development. The College responded by establishing a working party with representation from the specialist associations and the Raven Department of Education, reporting to the Education Board. A pilot scheme for continuing medical education accreditation within the College and an overview of the courses are being developed by the Department. A sessional tutor began to develop continuing medical education events in non-clinical areas that would complement the masterclasses prepared by the Hill Surgical Skills tutor, Alan Crockard (Fig 8.16), who was appointed Director of Education in 1998.

In 1998, the Senate determined that the scheme would be a joint effort of all four surgical Royal Colleges. The College agreed to fund and house its administration for a pilot phase of three years, and a new team was established within the External Affairs Department. The development of education courses continues to be the responsibility of the Raven Department of Education under the leadership of a sessional tutor. Masterclasses in surgical skills are offered, and from 1999 the programme of courses in continuing professional development is being broadened to reflect the needs of both established and aspiring consultants.

An International Role

The College's educational activities have changed its image among Fellows and surgical trainees: once viewed as an inward-looking, London-based organisation, the College is now seen to support its Fellows and trainees throughout the country. Over its first five years, the Raven Department of Education accounted for over 25 percent of College turnover, with a budget in excess of £4 million and more than 50 full-time members of staff.

In addition to its impact in the UK, its lead in education made the College an educational resource centre that now helps sister colleges and institutions in many countries all over the world. Over the last three years, the number of courses run by the College has grown rapidly in countries from Germany to South Africa. One particularly successful partnership is with the Royal Australasian College and the University of Western Australia to establish a skills centre in Perth. Another generous donation from Danny Hill has gone towards a unit that will be opened in May 2000.

CHAPTER 9

The Training Board: Improving Regional Structures

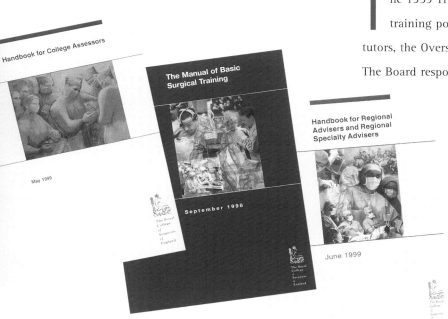

9.1 Training manuals published by the College

The 1959 Training Committee was superseded by the Training Board, which formulates training policies and oversees training, hospital recognition, the work of advisers and tutors, the Overseas Doctors' Training Committee and Women in Surgical Training (WIST). The Board responded with enthusiasm to the Calman training scheme (see also Chapter 10) by working with the Royal Surgical Colleges of Edinburgh, Glasgow and Ireland to introduce the MRCS/AFRCS and specialist FRCS examinations. Higher surgical training became an intercollegiate responsibility. At present, basic surgical training remains under the direction of individual Colleges, but the Colleges' intercollegiate committee standardises the requirements for basic surgical training throughout the British Isles.

The reorganisation of the senior house officer (SHO) programmes that began in 1996 shortened basic surgical training to two years. In 1998 the new MRCS examination was introduced, replacing the FRCS primary and final. The aim of basic surgical training is to provide a common core of training in the principles of surgery-in-general that will equip a trainee surgeon for higher surgical training in any surgical specialty.

The Hospital Recognition Committee is responsible for quinquennial reviews and numbering of all SHO posts. These visits ensure that every SHO post is numbered and offers trainees an opportunity to acquire the clinical skills common to all branches of surgery and to attain the attitudes, skills and knowledge needed at graduate level. The Training Board publishes a basic surgical training manual (the *Blue Book*) that defines the full details of this programme (Fig 9.1).

The visitors on the Hospital Recognition Committee comprise Council members, regional advisers, specialty representatives and interested surgeons prepared to give time to visit up to 20 hospitals in a particular region within a few months.

The College has always been reluctant to apply its ultimate sanction – withdrawal of recognition from posts at a hospital where the facilities or teaching are inadequate. Nevertheless, it is unusual for a visitor's report to be free of critical comment. Recognition is often for less than five years, and on condition that deficiencies are remedied before the next review.

In 1995 the College established a registration scheme for SHOs. Since 1998, trainees registered with the College as wishing to pursue a surgical career have been designated Affiliates of the College. Affiliate status is a precursor to membership and encourages trainees to establish an early and lasting association with the College by providing them with a 'passport' to its facilities. In 1998 the College appointed part-time advisers in careers and flexible training who are practising consultant surgeons in the National Health Service. They advise Affiliates on career options and opportunities at a time of intense competition for higher surgical training programmes.

Regional Advisers and Tutors

The day-to-day work of the Training Board is undertaken on its behalf by its network of regional advisers, regional specialty advisers and surgical tutors. They are the College's representatives throughout the country. Formally appointed by the College, and very often the 'public face' of the College in the locality, regional advisers and regional specialty advisers promote the standards of surgery. They co-ordinate training and talk to trainees, hospitals and Trusts on a wide spectrum of local training issues, as well as

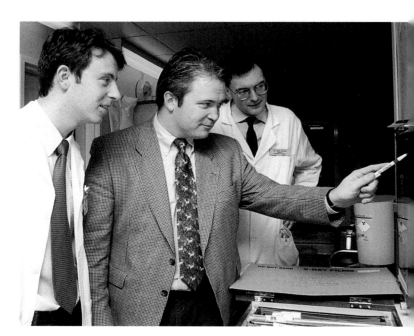

9.2 Consultant trainer with surgical trainees, St Mary's Hospital, 1999

9.2

provide a link between the College, universities and postgraduate deans. Surgical tutors play a key role in supporting trainees as they progress through their careers. These advisers and tutors do this important work without remuneration.

Since the early 1970s, there has been a surgical tutor in every acute hospital that has basic surgical trainees (Fig 9.2). At the outset, the tutor's responsibilities were to ensure that all SHOs received training and education appropriate to their needs, and were not merely used as underpaid assistants to provide care of patients at unsociable hours. The hard-pressed surgical tutor is often caught between the requirements of the trainees, the responsibilities of the College and the service demands of the employing Trust. The College continues to depend on the goodwill of the many surgeons who take on these responsibilities. Regional specialty advisers do not confine their attention to basic surgical trainees; they also have a wealth of responsibilities for higher surgical trainees.

The adviser's activities include arranging the appointment of surgical tutors in the hospitals in the region, taking part in the quinquennial visits organised by the Hospital Recognition Committee, and membership on the postgraduate medical and dental board that reviews overall training policy in the region. Specialty advisers are usually the driving force behind regional training schemes for specialist registrars.

The College's statutory responsibility in the appointment of consultants is exercised by regional specialty advisers who approve job descriptions for consultant posts. The job description will not be approved if the resources, support and facilities being offered to a new consultant are inadequate; if the job is not balanced in fixed and flexible sessions; or if insufficient time is allowed for operating lists, ward rounds, out-patient clinics, teaching, administration, research or on-call commitments. The regional specialty adviser ensures that a new consultant will not only be able to practise satisfactorily in the specialty, but will also be in a position to train the next generation of surgeons. This approval process remains the only external influence on the working arrangements for an incoming consultant surgeon.

Overseas Doctors' Training Scheme

Britain has a long tradition of welcoming medical and dental students as well as doctors and dentists from overseas who wish to pursue undergraduate or postgraduate education and

9.3 Sir David Innes Williams (b. 1919)

David Innes Williams qualified at University College Hospital and took resident surgical posts there from 1942. He served as urological surgeon at St Peter's Hospital from 1950 to 1978, and at the Hospital for Sick Children, Great Ormond Street, where he effectively founded the sub-specialty of paediatric urology. He was President of the British Association of Urological Surgeons 1976–78, Director of the British Postgraduate Medical Federation 1978–86, Pro Vice-Chancellor of the University of London 1985–87, Chairman of the Council of the Imperial Cancer Research Fund 1982–91, President of the British Medical Association 1988–89, and President of the Royal Society of Medicine 1990–92. He was Chairman of the Overseas Committee of the General Medical Council 1979–89. Sir David served on Council from 1974 to 1986, was Vice-President from 1983 to 1985, was awarded the Honorary Medal in 1987, and is the current Chairman of the Hunterian Trustees.

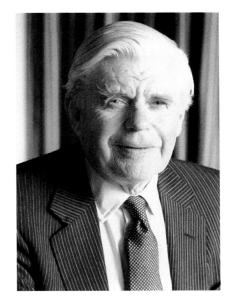

training, and who may stay on to seek employment in the UK. Study in the UK has made a major contribution to the health services of countries around the world, and has benefited both overseas doctors and the National Health Service. The College has always regarded the surgical training of doctors from overseas as complementary to the training of UK graduates, and often sponsors overseas doctors wishing to receive further surgical training in the UK.

In 1982 Sir David Innes Williams (Fig 9.3), then Director of the British Postgraduate Medical Federation and past Vice-President of the College, suggested that a National Overseas Doctors' Sponsorship Organisation be established. The scheme eventually adopted was based on his ideas, although

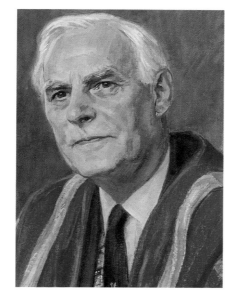

9.4 Sir Ian Todd (b. 1921)

Born into a family with medical connections going back several generations, from an early age Ian Todd had aspirations of becoming a surgeon. He trained at St Bartholomew's Hospital and in Canada; in due course, he practised surgery at Barts and St Mark's. Although he enjoyed clinical work, he became involved in administration, serving as Governor at Barts, President of the Medical Society of London, and as a member of Council before being elected President of the College. Throughout his career, he nurtured an interest in developing countries, and worked in many areas teaching, lecturing and operating, especially India and East Africa.

By June Mendoza

9.5 Professor Peter Bevan conducting a surgical workshop in Uganda, 1986

Peter Gilroy Bevan (b. 1922) served on Council from 1971 to 1983 and was Vice-President 1981–83. He was Chairman of the Board of Surgical Training for five years. Bevan's enthusiasm for surgical training manifested itself in his roles in starting anastomosis workshops and initiating the Overseas Doctors Training scheme. He organised the ODT scheme for three years, during which time 250 surgical training posts for overseas doctors were established. Bevan served also as Liaison Officer to Council, in which capacity he visited virtually every surgical department in England.

real progress could only be achieved following changes to the immigration laws in 1985. Sir Ian Todd (Fig 9.4), Chairman of the Council's Board of Surgical Training, used this opportunity to provide structured training programmes with a clear end-point.

Peter Bevan (Fig 9.5), Chairman, and David Evans, Vice-Chairman, promoted the Overseas Doctor Training scheme throughout England, Wales and Northern Ireland between September 1986 and January 1987. They also visited the United Arab Emirates, Riyadh, Khartoum and Cairo to discuss details with potential sponsors. Since 1987, the scheme has placed thousands of trainees from Argentina to Zimbabwe in recognised UK training posts for both basic and higher surgical training.

Overseas doctors were doubly sponsored. A UK consultant surgeon vouched for a trainee from a known overseas institution. The ODT scheme ensured that the trainee was of a sufficiently

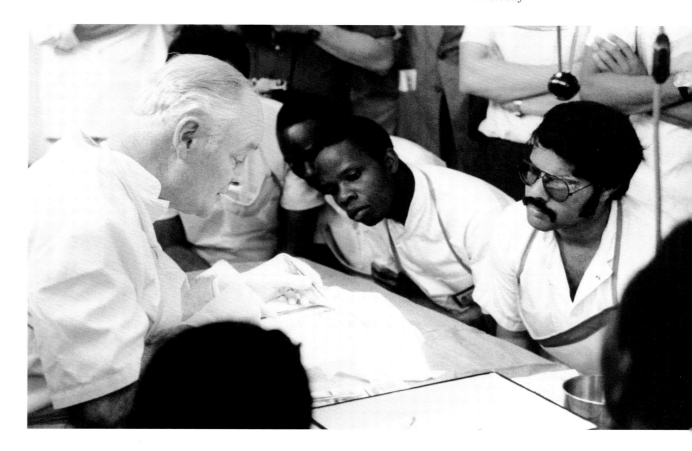

high calibre to fill the post on offer and confirmed to the General Medical Council the trainee's suitability for limited (temporary) registration; they were then exempt from the General Medical Council's Professional Linguistic Assessment Board examination. The ODT scheme assessed and monitored the trainee's performance and progress throughout the period of UK training.

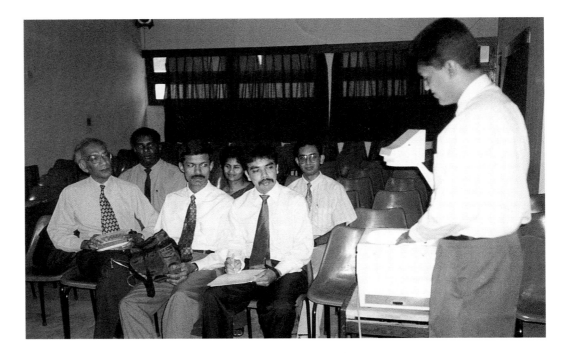

9.6 Review of candidates to participate in the pilot ODT scheme, 1999

The co-ordinator of the pilot scheme at the University of Colombo, Sri Lanka, is Professor Aluwihare, Chairman of the Department of Surgery, pictured seated at left.

The Calman changes to training and the resulting reduction in the training period at the SHO level led to a sharp decline in posts available to overseas doctors, particularly those seeking higher surgical training. However, most posts were already filled by UK trainees.

Single sponsorship, where the links with overseas institutions are directly with the College rather than between individual consultants, is currently favoured. A recent pilot scheme with the University of Colombo in Sri Lanka (Fig 9.6) involves specialist associations in the selection process and is addressing many perceived criticisms of the original scheme.

Women in Surgical Training

As long ago as 1985 women comprised half of the students entering medical schools, but only a small proportion of those women went on to become surgeons. The College found it necessary to consider how best it could respond to the under-representation of women.

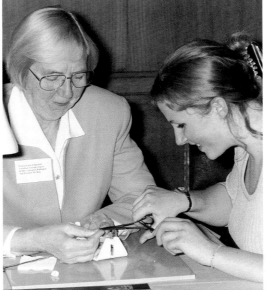

9.7 Professor Averil Mansfield at a College open evening

Professor Mansfield is a Professor of Surgery at St Mary's Hospital and a Vice-President of the College.

Professor Averil Mansfield (Fig 9.7) was given the task of chairing the WIST scheme when it was established in September 1991 as a joint initiative by the College and the Department of Health. The scheme is open to all women wishing to pursue a surgical career, and encourages them to enter surgical training (Fig 9.8). It also supports, advises and enables those women already in surgery to realise their professional goals.

In the first nine years after WIST's inception, the number of women surgical consultants doubled. There are now nearly 1,000 registered members of WIST, a network of 23 representatives providing advice and support to women in their respective region, and a directory of members prepared to give advice about particular issues.

The College was the first medical Royal College to join Opportunity Now (formerly Opportunity 2000), and in so doing opened a door for WIST to liaise with over 300 private and public sector organisations, covering over 25 percent of the UK workforce, that share similar concerns and aims. A business-led and business-driven campaign, Opportunity Now has a clear objective – to improve the quantity and quality of women's employment at all levels, based on ability. These aims and objectives are complementary to those of WIST and bode well for future collaboration.

9.8 Leela Kapila demonstrating laparoscopy for a WIST schools day

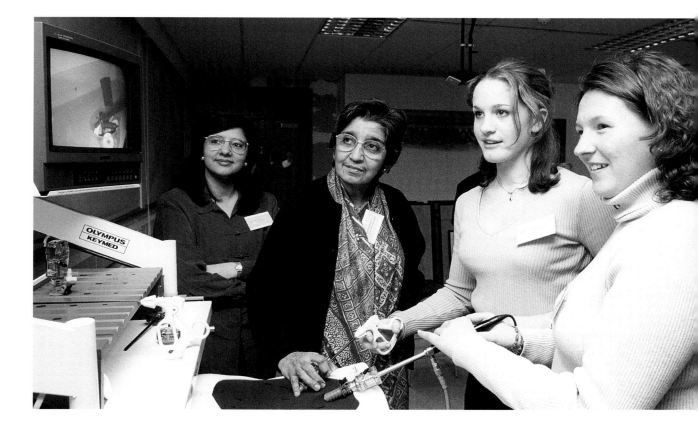

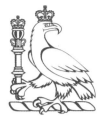

CHAPTER 10

Examinations:
A Decade *of* Reorganisation

A t the time of its foundation, the College was effectively the only body in England and Wales granting a practical surgical qualification. Theoretically, the medical graduates of Oxford and Cambridge and the Diplomates of the Royal College of Physicians of London were entitled to practise surgery, but they rarely did so. The *Apothecaries Act* of 1815 gave control of medical (as opposed to surgical) education in England (outside London) and Wales to the Society of Apothecaries. Within a few years it was common for candidates intending to enter general practice to sit both the Licentiate of the Society of Apothecaries (LSA) and the Membership of the Royal College of Surgeons (MRCS) examinations.

10.1 Examination papers from 1860

ROYAL COLLEGE OF SURGEONS OF ENGLAND.

THE

EXAMINATION PAPERS

AS SET FOR THE

PRELIMINARY LITERARY EXAMINATION

OF

CANDIDATES FOR THE DIPLOMA OF MEMBER

OF THE COLLEGE,

ON THE

26TH & 27TH JUNE, 1860;

CONDUCTED BY

EXAMINERS OF THE COLLEGE OF PRECEPTORS.

The College Charter of 1843 for the first time permitted the creation of Fellows. Fellowship of the Royal College of Surgeons (FRCS) was by nomination of Council in the first year; thereafter admission was by examination. Only 600 Fellows were admitted in the first year, and the dissatisfaction raised by this selectivity lasted half a century. The first examination took place 3–5 December 1844 and consisted of a two-hour written part of 48 anatomical questions; performance of an operation on a cadaver; and answering 30 oral questions on pathology, therapeutics and surgery. A high standard of general education was demanded; unless they had already passed an arts degree or equivalent, candidates for the Fellowship had to undergo an examination in Latin (Fig 10.1).

10.2 FRCS oral examination during
the Second World War

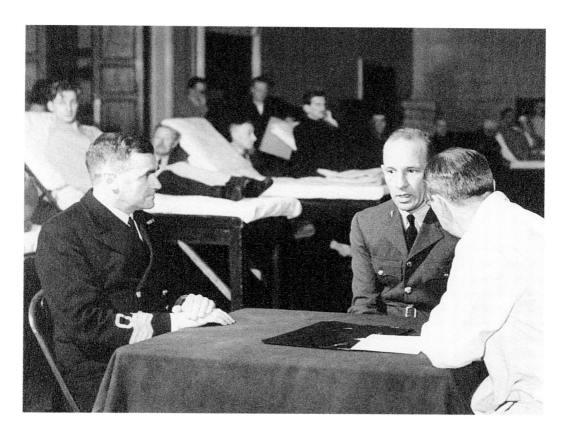

Anatomy and physiology became prominent features of the examination, and by 1867 the
Fellowship was divided into primary and pass sections. From 1870 the primary (encompassing
anatomy and physiology) was run by an independent examining board. Although there was
continuous concern and debate within the College about the content, format and purpose of
the examination, over the next 100 years the format remained unchanged (Figs 10.2 and 10.3).

10.3 **Successful candidates for the FRCS
standing before the Court of Examiners**

This photograph, taken in 1958, features Professor
Sir Roy Calne (see also Fig 6.14) standing at the end
nearest the camera. The Chairman of the Court at
the time was Arthur Dickson Wright.

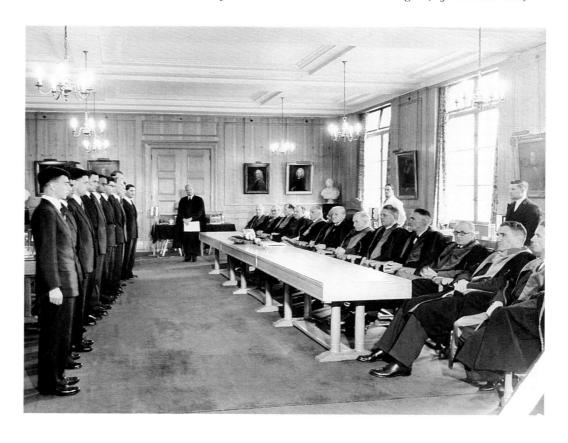

After the introduction of the National Health Service in 1948, the FRCS was an essential prerequisite to entering surgical training at the registrar level and for selection for senior registrar training. Recognition of a level of surgical competence suitable for consultant appointment lay not with the College but in the hands of each NHS Statutory Consultant Appointment Advisory Committee.

Specialist surgeons were particularly concerned about the absence of an advanced-level specialty assessment at the end of training, comparable to the American Board Examinations. In 1990, an event occurred that precipitated a complete re-evaluation of training programmes and examinations: an unexpected challenge to the legality of UK training certification with respect to European law.

As a result of the *Doctors' Directive* of 1975, all Colleges awarded a 'Certificate of Specialist Training' for the purposes of free movement between the countries of the European Union. This was granted without further examination or interview to anyone who had passed the FRCS examination and had worked for two years in approved registrar posts. However, UK Consultant Appointment Committees required a UK Certificate of Accreditation from the Specialist Advisory Committees, attesting that the trainee had satisfactorily completed a supervised training programme at the senior registrar level.

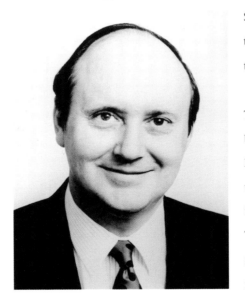

The administration in Brussels decided that the UK was setting two standards for specialists – the European Certificate (considered too low and too uncertain a standard for consultant appointment in the UK) and the UK Certificate of Accreditation. The European Commission informed the UK government that this was illegal and that they intended to institute infraction proceedings. The government responded by setting up a committee chaired by the Chief Medical Officer, Sir Kenneth Calman, to review UK specialist training (Fig 10.4), and his report was issued in 1993.

Knowing this was likely to happen, the surgical Colleges had already formulated their views on surgical training and incorporated them into Calman's report: surgical training should be divided into two periods – the first should last two years and concentrate on the core knowledge and skills required of all surgeons regardless of specialty, and the second should last five or six years and cover specialist training, subspecialty training and, if possible, some exposure to surgical research. The first two years were to be in the senior

10.4 Sir Kenneth Calman (b. 1941)

Following house jobs, Kenneth Calman went to the Department of Surgery in Glasgow with clinical interests in general surgery, vascular surgery and transplantation. In 1972, he was the MRC Clinical Research Fellow at the Chester Beatty Research Institute in London and in 1974 returned to Glasgow as Professor of Oncology. He remained in that post for ten years developing particular interests in nutrition, chemotherapy, cancer education, counselling and patient support groups. In 1984 he became Dean of Postgraduate Medicine and Professor of Postgraduate Medical Education at the University of Glasgow. In 1989 he was appointed Chief Medical Officer at the Scottish Home and Health Department and in September 1991 became Chief Medical Officer in the Department of Health in London. In 1998 he was appointed Vice-Chancellor and Warden of the University of Durham.

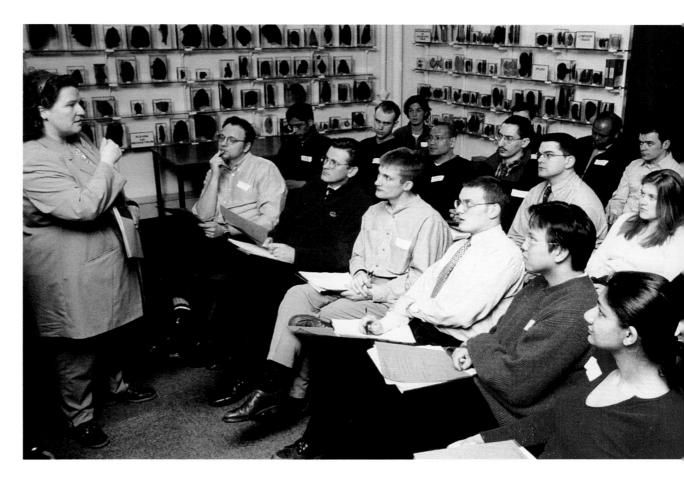

10.5 A study day for the STEP course for the MRCS

house officer grade, and the next five or six years in a new grade called specialist registrar – an amalgamation of the old registrar and senior registrar grades.

The supervision, teaching and testing of the specialist registrar grades were already well controlled by the Specialist Advisory Committees, whose intercollegiate examination needed only minor revision. Teaching and supervision of basic surgery in general and its testing at the end, however, needed drastic reformation. The newly established Raven Department of Education immediately set about developing a distance learning (*STEP*) course to correspond with the syllabus for basic surgical training (Fig 10.5).

If the intercollegiate specialist FRCS Diploma was to be an exit qualification at the end of higher surgical training, a new diploma was needed to signify completion of basic surgical training. The appropriate qualification of MRCS was already part of the Conjoint Diploma (LRCP, MRCS). Changing this required an amendment by Parliament of the 1983 *Medical Act*. Lord McColl (a past Council Member) successfully brought a Private Member's Bill before Parliament in May 1991.

Upon approval by the Privy Council, the Conjoint Diploma became LRCP, LRCS, releasing the MRCS as the diploma for basic surgical training. The title 'Fellow' was reserved for those who successfully completed their specialty training and passed the relevant intercollegiate specialty examination. The significance and status of the Fellowship as the highest honour to be awarded by the College was restored.

The New Members

Basic surgical training is designed to provide broad exposure to surgical practice and the acquisition of general surgical knowledge and applied basic sciences. Surgical attachments must include a six-month period in each of four different specialties, of which at least two must have a significant emergency workload. The MRCS written examination comprises two

10.6 MRCS candidate undergoing the clinical examination

Photograph by Wayne Perry

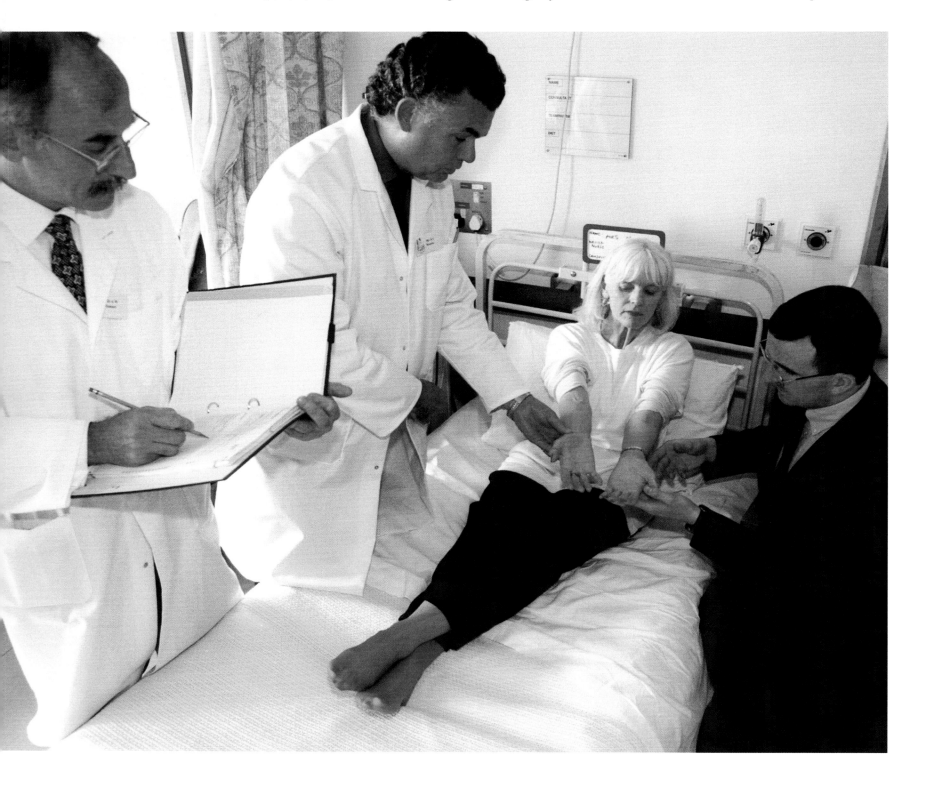

MCQ papers, one based on the contents of the core and one on systems modules of the published syllabus. The clinical examination assesses candidates on clinical problems and their communication skills (Fig 10.6). After passing the clinical examination, candidates attend the College for viva voce examinations, when the candidate's logbook is examined. Successful candidates are presented to the President as full Members of the College on Diplomates Day (Fig 10.7).

The new Members have all the rights of existing Fellows: they may vote in Council elections, stand for Council and use the courtesy title 'Mr' or 'Miss'. The first new-style Members were admitted by Council after the first examination in June 1998.

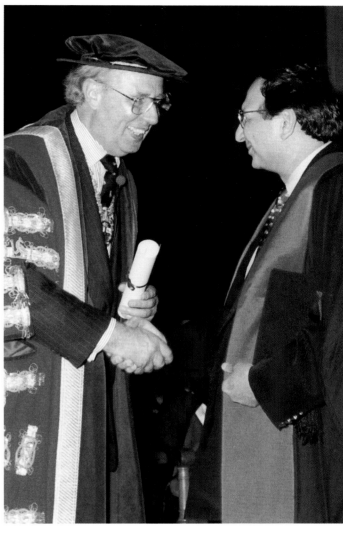

The New Fellows

The five or six years of specialist registrar training is a hands-on apprenticeship supplemented by personal audit, outcome assessment, specialist courses, conferences and regular reviews by each hospital and regional training committee, culminating in the intercollegiate specialist exam. The duration of this training was planned and calculated before the recent rigorous implementation of European Union working hours, and if these restrictions seriously reduce the clinical experience of the trainees, training periods may have to be extended.

With the present system of training, supervision, continuous assessment and examinations, the College believes that it is fulfilling the requirement of its Charter – the maintenance of the highest possible surgical standards – by ensuring that surgeons are trained to the highest level possible before beginning their consultant career. The College is well aware that advances in modern medicine demand that all training programmes and examinations be constantly reviewed and updated to meet the needs of the day. While the old FRCS served its purpose for 150 years, the present system provides an excellent foundation to take us into the new millennium.

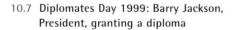

10.7 Diplomates Day 1999: Barry Jackson, President, granting a diploma

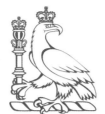

CHAPTER 11

Research and Audit: Promoting Effectiveness in Practice

11.1 Professor Sir Peter Morris (b. 1934)

First Chairman of the Research Board and the Nuffield Professor of Surgery, Director of the Oxford Transplant Centre, Oxford University and Fellow of the Royal Society.

In the early 1990s, the advent of molecular biology and an increasing need for high technology equipment in many areas of research meant that the role of a research institute independent of a university environment was difficult to sustain; in addition, the separation from hospitals was believed to be inappropriate. An external review commissioned under the Chairmanship of Sir Michael Peckham convinced Council to wind down its support for research within the College and to move the clinically active units to an appropriate medical

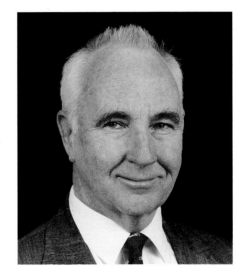

school. The Biophysics Unit was moved to the Institute of Child Health and the Dental Sciences Department to the King's College School of Medicine and Dentistry. Both units are thriving in their new clinical environments, and their chairs continue to be funded by the College.

The question then arose, 'What should the College's involvement in research be, if any?' The President, Sir Norman Browse (see also Fig 8.1), put to Council a case for establishing a research fellowship scheme. His argument was that all surgeons in surgical training should have the opportunity to spend one year in a structured research programme. If the Department of Health would not fund this, then the College should establish research fellowships. Council agreed, and Sir Peter Morris (Fig 11.1) was appointed Chairman of the new Research Board to establish the Research Fellowship Scheme. Later he undertook responsibility for the Surgical Epidemiology and Audit Unit created by Brendan Devlin (Fig 11.2).

11.2 Brendan Devlin (1932–1998)

Educated in Dublin, Brendan Devlin studied public administration and political science before medicine. He joined the surgical rotation at St Thomas's and then accepted an appointment to Stockton in 1970; four years later he was responsible for commissioning the new North Tees General Hospital, which he put on the map by his teaching and publications. He chaired the British Standards Institution Committee on Stoma Appliances, the DHSS Specialist Panel on Stoma Care and the British Colostomy Society. He established a multi-centre audit of groin hernia surgery, which led to the publication of guidelines and a classic textbook on the subject. His work in establishing the Confidential Enquiry into Peri-operative Deaths (CEPOD) set new standards for national audit and had a profound effect on management systems and patient care. Elected to Council in 1986, he set up and chaired the Clinical Audit and Quality Assurance Committee. As Chairman of the Examination Committee, he was active in bringing about the long overdue reforms of the FRCS.

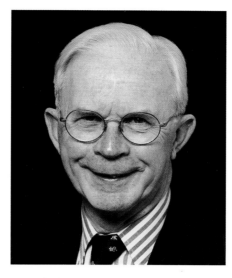

The first aim was to establish a number of research fellowships. The scheme started with endowments already designated for research activities. In the first year of planning, approaches for donations were made to the Fellows as well as to a variety of companies. These donations and College endowments allowed the scheme to be launched in 1993 with the advertisement of 15 Research Fellowships. By 1996, the number had risen to 75 in a wide variety of fields including plastic surgery, transplantation biology, orthopaedics, cancer, neurobiology, vascular physiology and molecular biology. Today the College awards more than 30 Research Fellowships each year.

A criticism has been made that one-year fellowships do not provide the trainee with adequate time to undertake a good research project. However, the Research Board tries to ensure that approved projects provide both training opportunities and skilled supervision for the Fellows (Figs 11.3–5). Many Fellowships are awarded at the end of a one- or two-year period of research to allow the trainees to complete their projects. In many cases, after one year with a College Research Fellowship, trainees find funding from elsewhere to continue their research. Despite initial scepticism within the academic surgical community, the Fellowships have rapidly become highly prized by trainees, and the number of applications from Members and Fellows of the College increases each year.

11.3 Research Fellow in orthopaedics with his supervisor in Newcastle

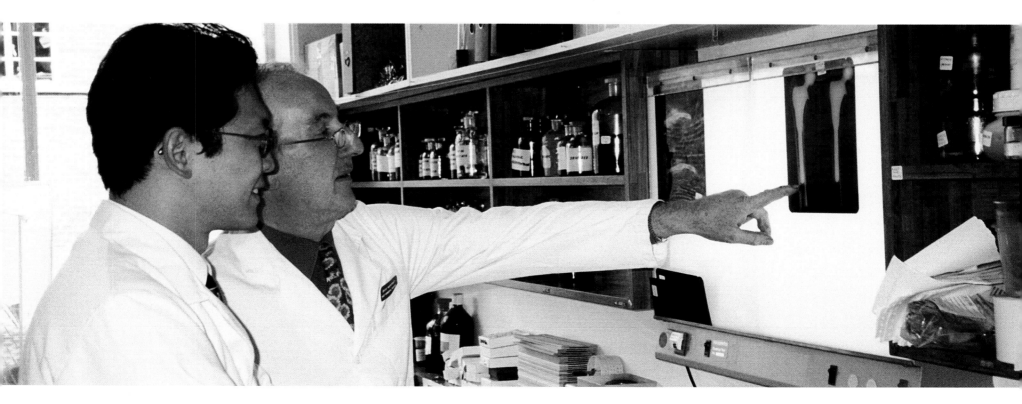

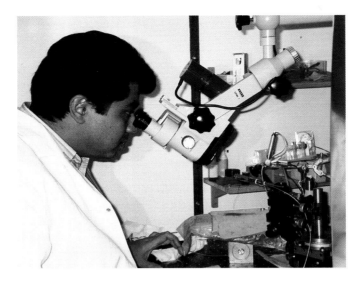

11.4 Research Fellow in otorhinolaryngology
in Brighton

When the Medical Research Council expressed concern about the declining numbers of young surgeons applying for Medical Research Council Training Fellowships, the Board successfully negotiated with that body joint funding for three-year training fellowships. Since the first two awards in 1996, Fellowships have been awarded every six months. This scheme has gone from strength to strength, and although initiated as a pilot scheme, has been outstandingly successful in attracting the best young academic surgeons. Many of the successful applicants, in what must be the most competitive field for research fellowships in the UK, are holders of an initial one-year College Research Fellowship.

Two other types of fellowship have been introduced: a small number of two-year research fellowships often jointly funded with another charitable body, and a small number of three-year fellowships for which departments bid, rather than individuals. These have proved very successful and the College hopes to raise more funding by this means in future.

In 1996, owing to concern about the difficulty met by newly appointed consultants in obtaining research support immediately after their appointment, the Research Board established a small number of pump-priming grants of up to £20,000 each awarded for specific research

11.5 Research Fellows in general surgery
with their supervisor in Liverpool

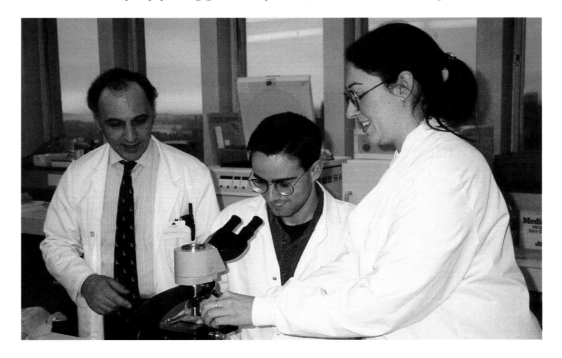

projects by consultants within three years of appointment. The response was overwhelming: the budget was increased from £100,000 for five projects to £138,000 for eight projects in the first year. This initiative continues to be enormously popular.

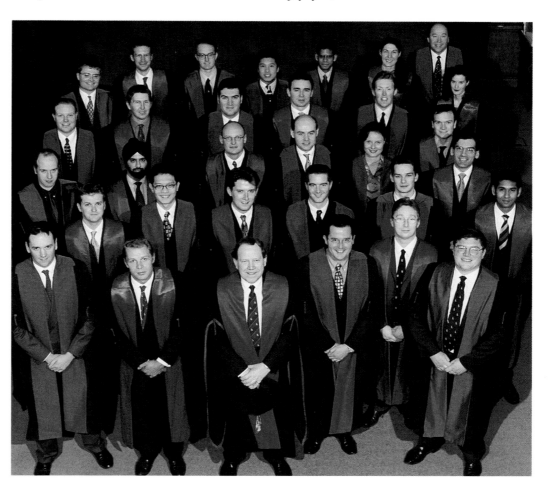

11.6 **1998 Research Fellows with Board Chairman Professor Peter Bell**

After six years, the Research Board reaffirmed the College's commitment to supporting research in surgery in a substantial way. The College has funded over 180 Research Fellowships since the scheme started and is contributing over £1 million per year to the programme. The scheme has a high profile among Fellows and the public, and has generated much goodwill towards the College. At the end of 1997, Sir Peter Morris handed over the Chairmanship of the Board to Professor Peter Bell, who continues to expand the scheme (Fig 11.6).

From Audit to Clinical Effectiveness

From John Hunter's time, surgeons have used a variety of methods to ensure that they achieve the best results from a particular procedure. Hunter pioneered routine post-operative monitoring and not only recorded the outcome of the operation but shared the results with colleagues by presenting them at small meetings and publishing them (Fig 11.7). Since Hunter's day some modification has been required as surgical practice evolves. It is no longer sufficient for a surgeon to scrutinise his or her own work. Modern surgical audit uses methods from other disciplines. For example, techniques of quality control are adapted from industrial models, experts in health services research help design the studies, and statisticians provide advice on

Lithotomy.

A Child was cut, and had the common treatment before and after the Operation. The stone was small. The second day, was dressed warm, and the water came through the wound, which was the first time of making water. At night had a shivering fit which they say is common, especially if the water does not come away; but this was not the Case here as he had made water freely about half an hour before the fit Second day pretty well. Fourth day, feverish, would have been bled if it had continued till night. Fifth day, pretty well. Sixth day. The water came the right way. Seventh day the same; and pretty regular Stools all the time. The 8th 9th 10th and 11th the same. More water coming the right way. 12th The wound touched with blue-stone, dressed with lint. Went on better and better till the wound healed on the 20th — This Case is kept merely on account of the Shivering Fit.

11.7 John Hunter's casebook

Hunter's casebooks demonstrate his eagerness to diagnose and then document his patients' conditions in detail. For instance, he describes five lithotomies (a hazardous procedure to remove stones from the urinary bladder) performed over the course of the 1720s. Following each operation, Hunter carefully recorded the outcome.

In two of the cases in his casebook, the patients were children (numbers 256 and 257). For the first of these, Hunter wrote, '10th (post-operative day) better, and continued so till he went out'. Undoubtedly a good result. The second case proved as successful, 'he went out well'. Some of the adults, however, sustained complications. In one patient who had 'for some time the symptoms of the stone and at last suppression of urine (case 259)', the outcome was poor: 'She went to the country and stayed two months; I then saw her at the hospital: she was better, but on walking, the water dropped from her'.

the most appropriate methods of analysis. Once the results are known, they are packaged in a way that is easily understood before being distributed to interested parties.

Ernest Avery Codman, a surgeon at Harvard University, was the first to incorporate modern techniques into the process now known as surgical audit. In a lecture delivered to the Philadelphia County Medical Society just before the First World War, he stated:

> We must formulate some method of hospital report showing as nearly as possible what are the results of treatment obtained at different institutions. This report must be made out and published by each hospital in a uniform manner, so that comparison will be possible. With such a report as a starting point, those interested can begin to ask questions as to management and efficiency.

Initially, Codman's efforts to bring industrial standards of quality control to bear on medicine met with ridicule. Now, he is seen as a visionary. Since Codman's time many others have contributed to the development of modern surgical audit. In 1984, Brendan Devlin, John Lumley and John Lunn introduced the Confidential Enquiry into Peri-operative Deaths (CEPOD), a nationwide survey that examines the causes of death following an operation. CEPOD is now a core activity funded by central government, and the identical format has been adopted in several other countries. The National CEPOD started in 1989 as a direct development of the original study.

The National CEPOD demonstrated that collaborative studies in which surgeons pool data and share experiences can be helpful. By taking a collaborative approach, it is possible to generate powerful data sets containing the results of many thousands of operations performed over a specified period of time. Surgeons who have carried out a small number of a particular operation can study the results of the same surgery performed in other institutions – by different surgeons and on different patients. This process hailed the start of collaborative or global audit – a process that in the 1990s became known as comparative audit.

Formalising Collaborative Surgical Studies

The first collaborative studies were carried out by groups of enthusiastic surgeons united by their love for computers. A small number of surgeons in the late 1980s recorded details of their operations on software known as Surgical Administration Systems. The Micromed™ and the Dunnfile™ user groups were the first comparative auditors. David Dunn (of Dunnfile™) was the pioneer in this field (Fig 11.8). This process was formalised by the College with the Surgical Epidemiology and Audit Unit in 1990 under Brendan Devlin, who sought to involve as many surgeons and specialties as possible in comparative audit. Happily, he achieved his goal. Before Devlin died at the end of 1998, he was able to report that nearly 3,000 surgeons from nearly every surgical specialty had contributed complete data on over 60,000 operations. This process continues and, like CEPOD, has been adopted by other related organisations.

Some issues require separate, comprehensive and carefully designed studies in order to be addressed adequately. The results from these studies have been used, in combination with the relevant literature and expert opinion, to generate clinical practice guidelines intended for wide distribution and adoption by specialist associations.

In 1995, Council asked Sir Richard Doll to chair a strategic review of the College's future policy for surgical audit. The group consulted widely and in December 1996 published its report, in which Doll made the following recommendations:

- The unit should continue its commitment in educating and training surgeons in matters of surgical audit; development of sound audit procedures; setting the agenda for national clinical audit in the field of surgery and encouraging both research and discussion that might lead to the publication of clinical guidelines.

- This commitment should be implemented through a ten-year programme in collaboration with an academic partner.

- The new unit should have a scientific base, a more precise focus and closer links with surgical developments.

- The new unit should have a core staff that would provide the necessary continuity and be able to provide the surgical and methodological expertise required.

- The unit should be renamed so as to reflect its wider remit.

11.8 David Christy Dunn (1939–1998)

David Dunn was a pioneer in comparative audit and President of the Association of Endoscopic Surgeons of Great Britain and Ireland. Appointed a consultant general surgeon to Addenbrooke's in 1974, Dunn took up endoscopic surgery which was then in its infancy, seeing the potential for converting major surgery into a short stay procedure. He directed the College Comparative Audit Service set up to identify problems in this area; this in turn led to the development of recognised training programmes.

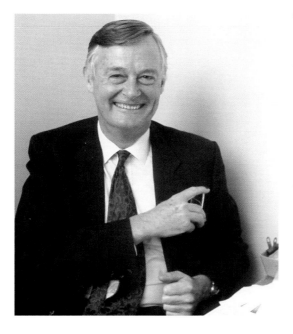

The Director of the new Clinical Effectiveness Unit, Barnaby Reeves, is supported by an advisory committee comprising representatives from the surgical specialties and reports directly to the College's Research Board. The Clinical Effectiveness Unit is a joint unit academically linked with the Health Services Research Unit at the London School of Hygiene and Tropical Medicine headed by Professor Nick Black.

The College is thus in a unique position to address issues of surgical audit, quality, clinical effectiveness and clinical governance. A team has been assembled with the required multidisciplinary expertise, appropriate links to a first class academic unit and, perhaps most importantly, a mechanism to encourage a dialogue with all the surgical specialties.

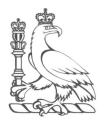

CHAPTER 12

Faculty *of* Anaesthetists

12.1 Sir Humphry Davy (1778–1829)

Davy experimented with nitrous oxide on himself and his literary friends. They described their feelings as: *'Highly pleasurable thrilling, particularly in the chest and extremities...objects became dazzling and my hearing more acute...sublime emotions connected with highly vivid ideas.'* (Davy) *'I immediately laughed...a sensation perfectly new and delightful.'* (Robert Southey) *'More unmingled pleasure than I had ever before experienced.'* (Samuel Taylor Coleridge).

Davy concluded: *'As nitrous oxide appears capable of destroying physical pain, it may probably be used with advantage during surgical operations.'* In spite of his suggestion, nearly half a century was to elapse before anaesthesia was used for this purpose. Davy must have known of the agony of surgery, for he had been apprenticed to John Bingham Borlase, surgeon of Penzance. However, he changed direction and went on to become the first President of the Royal Institution and never followed up any of his early work on nitrous oxide.

Painting by T Phillips [Courtesy National Portrait Gallery, London]

12.2 Henry Hill Hickman (1800–1830)

A Shropshire general practitioner, he must be credited with having tried hard to produce surgical anaesthesia. He tried carbon dioxide in animals and achieved short periods of oblivion to painful stimuli, which he called 'suspended animation', followed by full recovery. Unfortunately, what he was really producing was brief periods of reversible asphyxia. Although Davy's work on nitrous oxide had been published in 1800, there is no evidence that Hickman knew of this and his attempts to publicise his findings were, perhaps fortunately, unsuccessful.

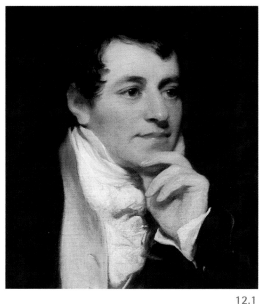

12.1

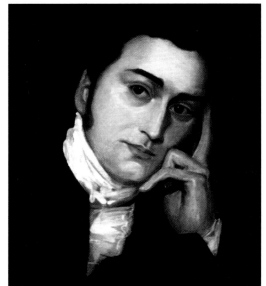

12.2

Although in 1799 Humphry Davy (Fig 12.1) observed the anaesthetic effect of nitrous oxide on himself when afflicted with toothache, his discovery was virtually disregarded, as was the suggestion, believed to have been made by his pupil Michael Faraday, that the same effect could be produced by ether vapour. Unfortunately, neither Davy nor Faraday took the investigations further, but a young Shropshire doctor named Henry Hill Hickman (Fig 12.2) continued the pursuit of painless surgery. He qualified as a Member of the College in 1820, and his experiments producing anaesthesia in animals using carbon dioxide were partially successful. If he had known of Davy's experience and used nitrous oxide he might today be known as the discoverer of surgical anaesthesia. Instead, his attempts to gain recognition for his work failed and he died a disappointed man.

12.3 Theatre poster

'Laughing gas' was inhaled to the point of excitement and participants encouraged to make fools of themselves for the entertainment of spectators.

Meanwhile, ether and nitrous oxide were used in a small way for theatrical entertainment (Fig 12.3) and as recreational drugs. In the 1840s 'laughing gas' parties and 'ether frolics' were the rage both in Britain and in the United States. Not until 1845 did the young dentist Horace Wells in Hartford, Connecticut, show that the inhalation of nitrous oxide could allow operations to be performed without pain. When another dentist, William Thomas Green Morton, used ether for an operation at the Massachusetts General Hospital in Boston, the news spread quickly to London. Within weeks, Robert Liston (Fig 12.4) had successfully used ether for an amputation of the leg. It was soon adapted for use in childbirth, until James Young

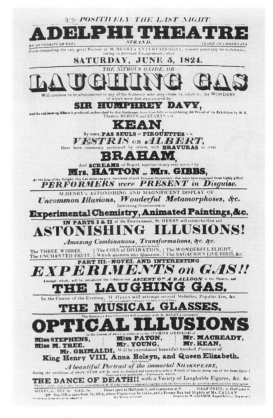

12.3

Simpson in Edinburgh showed that chloroform was better. Inevitably, objections were raised: some obstetricians thought pain was in some way a protective mechanism, and some people believed that the Bible required pain in childbirth – the legacy of Eve's sin in the garden of Eden. However, when news leaked out that John Snow (Fig 12.5) had administered chloroform to the Queen at the birth of Prince Leopold in 1853, anaesthesia began to become respectable.

Within a few years, several doctors began to specialise in the new field (Fig 12.6). Among the first of these specialists, Snow published a scholarly textbook on anaesthesia entitled *On the inhalation of ether vapour* in 1847, remarkably soon after ether's first use as an anaesthetic.

12.4 Robert Liston (1774–1847)

Professor of surgery at University College Hospital, Liston became the first surgeon in Europe to perform a capital (major) operation under anaesthesia, when he amputated Frederick Churchill's leg on 21 December 1846. A painless dental extraction under ether had been performed two days earlier by James Robinson at 14 Gower Street, not far from University College Hospital.

12.5 John Snow (1813–1858)

The eldest son of a Yorkshire farmer, Snow was one of the first students to enter the Newcastle-upon-Tyne Medical School in 1832. Later he walked to London to study at the Hunterian School of Anatomy. He became the first specialist anaesthetist and was appointed to St George's Hospital. He gave chloroform to Queen Victoria for her seventh pregnancy, and when she went into labour for her eighth pregnancy, she demanded to have 'that blessed chloroform' again. When Snow arrived, he found Prince Albert had already started to administer it to the Queen on his handkerchief. Snow was a brilliant pioneer not only in anaesthesia, but also in epidemiology. He shortened an outbreak of cholera in Soho by removing the handle of the Broad Street water pump, having deduced from the spread of the disease that it must be a water-borne infection. He died aged 45 from phthisis and nephritis.

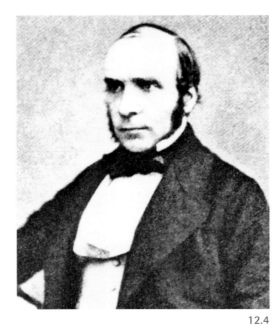

12.4

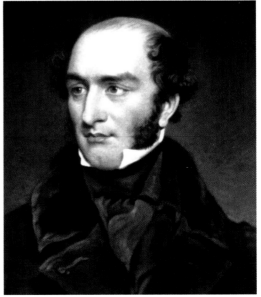

12.5

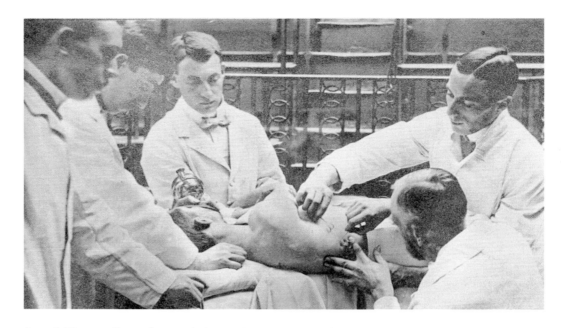

12.6

A typical scene, probably in the 1890s, showing an operation under anaesthesia by Sir Rickman Godlee at University College Hospital. The theatre was the site of Liston's first operation under anaesthesia in 1846.

[Courtesy Royal Society of Medicine]

12.7 Joseph Thomas Clover (1825–1882)

Born in Aylsham, Norfolk, Clover apprenticed to a surgeon in Norwich before proceeding to University College Hospital. He became Fellow of the College, intending to practise as a surgeon, but after Snow's early death, became the leading anaesthetist in London. He designed apparatus both for anaesthesia and for surgery.

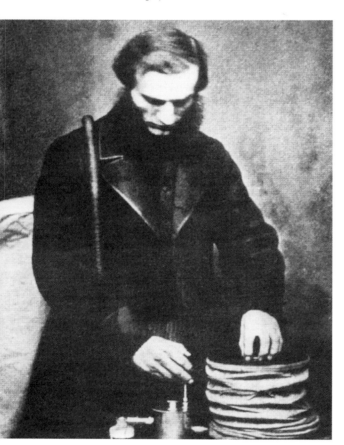

12.8 Clover's ether inhaler of 1877

Note the similar apparatus used in Godlee's operation (Fig 12.6). Clover laid great stress on using apparatus that gave a measurable concentration of vapour rather than relying on the guesswork of pouring it on to a cloth.

[Courtesy Association of Anaesthetists of Great Britain and Ireland]

Joseph Thomas Clover (Fig 12.7) designed many pieces of anaesthetic apparatus (Fig 12.8). He worked with Sir Henry Thompson, the pioneer of lithotripsy. (It was Clover who suggested that, after the stone had been crushed, the fragments should be sucked out of the bladder and he devised a special bulb for the purpose; Thompson, however, was slow to take up the idea.)

Cocaine, long known to native South Americans as a stimulant and euphoriant drug, was employed by Carl Koller of Vienna in 1884 as a topical local anaesthetic in the eye. William Stewart Halsted in New York injected it into nerve trunks to provide regional analgesia, not at first realising its potential for toxicity and addiction.

By the end of the century London could boast sufficient anaesthetists that they regarded their science as a legitimate specialty, and in 1893 they founded the world's first Society of Anaesthetists. An editorial in the *Lancet* welcomed the Society as a sound development, though added that if anaesthetists did not make progress now, they would have only themselves to blame. In 1908, the anaesthetists merged themselves into the Section of Anaesthetics of the Royal Society of Medicine. There were three women doctors among the founder members; thus were the anaethetists one of the first medical societies to accept women.

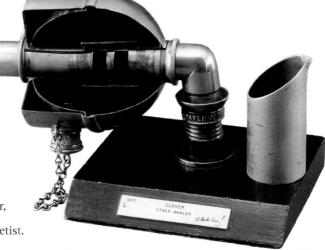

The First World War expanded the scope of surgery and inspired a young army doctor, Ivan Magill (Fig 12.9), to become an anaesthetist. His best-known innovation was to facilitate endotracheal intubation, designing his own equipment and constructing his tubes from soft rubber, which, being stored in a round biscuit tin and left to vulcanise in the sulphurous London atmosphere, acquired the

12.8

12.9 Sir Ivan Magill (1888-1986)

As an army doctor at Sidcup, Kent, Magill devised means of maintaining the airway for the new specialty of reconstructive surgery of the face and jaws. While not the originator of tracheal intubation, he designed apparatus that enabled the technique to be mastered by all anaesthetists. He developed the art of blind nasal intubation in the pre-curare days, when it could take longer and required deeper anaesthesia to manipulate a laryngoscope than was needed for the operation itself. Circuits, laryngoscopes and tubes of his design are still in use today.

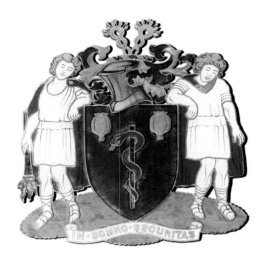

12.10 First coat of arms of the Association of Anaesthetists

Note that anaesthetists can make the flames from a burning torch flow downwards!

necessary stiffness and curvature. He then cut them to length and sanded the ends down to the required smoothness.

Magill was also convinced of the need for a diploma in anaesthetics. Because its charter would not permit him to set one up within the Section of Anaesthetics, Magill recommended the formation of a new organisation. Thus, in 1932 the Association of Anaesthetists of Great Britain and Ireland was founded (Fig 12.10). Two years later, this Association approached the Royal College of Surgeons about adding anaesthetics to the diplomas they already administered. Progress was speedy, and 17 months later the first examination was held for 54 candidates, of whom 46 passed.

During the 1930s, anaesthesia continued advancing steadily, and the Diploma sufficed for this period. However, the 1940s changed all this. Three apparently unconnected events launched anaesthesia on its rise from a skilled craft to a scientific discipline and raised the status of both the practice and the practitioners: the introduction of curare in 1942, the Second World War 1939–1945, and the National Health Service in 1948.

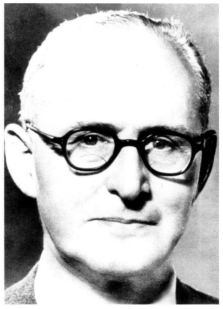

12.9

A New Concept – Curare is Introduced

For centuries native Central Americans had dipped the tips of their arrows in curare, which paralysed prey upon impact. In 1942 British anaesthetists readily perceived that, because of its paralysing effects on all muscles, curare offered the potential for a conceptual advance, opening the way for safer, more controllable anaesthesia. However, dealing with a paralysed patient unable to breathe demanded a knowledge of applied physiology that did not then exist. To exploit the full potential of curare, anaesthetists had to go back to the laboratory; in the following decades research efforts into the application of basic science to anaesthesia proliferated rapidly.

Curare provided the intellectual challenge that turned anaesthesia from a craft into a science. Using curare gave anaesthetists experience that increased demand for their skills to treat respiratory failure outside the operating theatre, and led ultimately to the development of intensive care units. It also gave rise to the concept of second-to-second observation and control that has been anaesthesia's greatest contribution to medicine. But much more than scientific advance was needed; in particular, more anaesthetists with the time and ability to conduct further research.

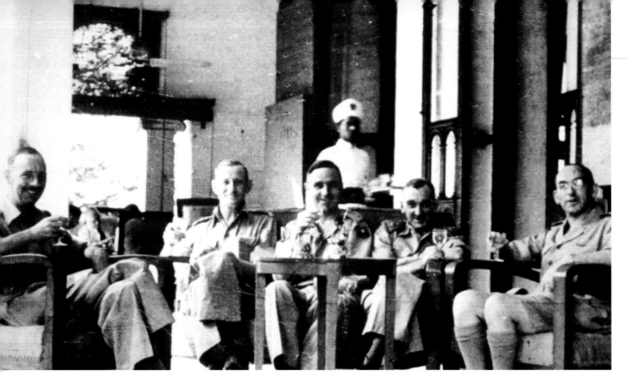

12.11 Army anaesthetists W McConnell, Vernon Frederick Hall, K Ashworth, TAB Harris and Victor Goldman in India, 1944

These doctors were among the few experienced anaesthetists in the army and were responsible for training many more for the field surgical units. All went on to have distinguished post-war careers in the National Health Service. Hall was a founder member of the Faculty of Anaesthetists in 1948.

[Courtesy Vernon Frederick Hall]

12.12 Archibald Marston (1891–1962)

Anaesthetist at Guy's Hospital and first Dean of the Faculty of Anaesthetists.

[Courtesy Royal College of Anaesthetists]

Armed Forces Anaesthetists

In the Second World War, the Royal Army Medical Corps created large numbers of mobile surgical teams to treat casualties near the front line. There were plenty of surgeons but anaesthetists were few. Before the war, any doctor was expected to administer anaesthetics; surgeons, for financial reasons, usually asked the patient's general practitioner to do it.

As a result, specialist anaesthetists were edged out and struggled to make a living. The Army, therefore, had to train its own anaesthetists and developed a cadre of enthusiastic teachers (Fig 12.11). When their young trainees returned to civilian life ready to continue with their new specialty, they sought permanent posts that previously had not existed.

Post-war Britain was a changed place, not least with the Labour government's plans for a free health service. In 1947, the only antibiotics were sulphonamides and penicillin; tuberculosis killed 23,000 people each year; and a recent poliomyelitis epidemic had killed 500, mostly young people. The pre-war voluntary hospitals had run out of funds.

The National Health Service

The new National Health Service provided a great opportunity for anaesthetists. The nationalised hospitals needed full-time, salaried staff and provided posts for the anaesthetists who had been trained by the armed forces for war-time service.

At the beginning, only the three Royal Colleges (Physicians, Surgeons and Obstetricians) were consulted by government; possibly it was believed that no other medical staff would attain consultant status, but would remain hospital medical officers with lower status and pay. Anaesthetists, along with pathologists, radiologists and other specialties, were left out of government consultation. The leading anaesthetists realised that in order to gain recognition they must show solid evidence of academic excellence, for which purpose the Faculty of Anaesthetists was founded.

The Founding of the Faculty

During the war, The Royal College of Surgeons had co-opted to its Council an anaesthetist nominated by the Association. Their choice of Archibald Marston of Guy's Hospital was excellent (Fig 12.12), for he already enjoyed both the friendship and respect of the College President, Lord Webb-Johnson.

12.12

With nationalised healthcare a certainty, Marston and Webb-Johnson moved quickly, believing that for anaesthetists to gain consultant status, they must have an academic organisation and an examination of Fellowship standard. The idea was backed by Sir Henry Souttar, a surgeon who strongly favoured the creation of faculties within the College and had been instrumental in the formation of the Faculty of Dental Surgery the year before (see also Fig 15.24). Marston also had support from Bernard Johnson of the Middlesex Hospital. Together they persuaded the Association to approach the College about setting up a Faculty within the College. In February 1948, it was agreed to establish the Faculty of Anaesthetists. Its dean would be elected by Council, and there would be 21 board members in addition to the President and Vice-Presidents ex officio. The first priority was to develop a Fellowship examination.

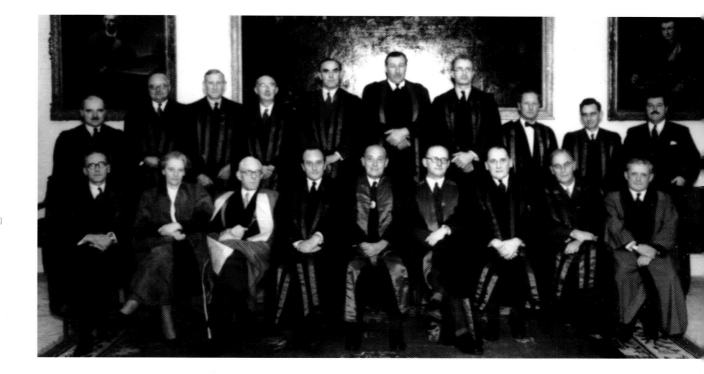

12.13 The first Board of Faculty of Anaesthetists, March 1948

Front row, left to right: John Humphrey Thornton Challis, Katherine Georgina Lloyd-Williams, Edgar Stanley Rowbotham, Bernard Johnson (Vice-Dean), Archibald Daniel Marston (Dean), Ivan Whiteside Magill, George Edwards, Christopher Langton-Hewer, Reginald Ernest Pleasance. Back row: Thomas Cecil Gray, Frankis Tilney Evans, Vernon Frederick Hall, Bernard Leo Salmon Murtagh, William Alexander Low, Ronald Francis Woolmer, Geoffrey SW Organe, Edgar Alexander Pask, William F Davis. Absent: John Gillies, Robert Reynolds Macintosh, Alec Hugh Musgrove.

[Courtesy Royal College of Anaesthetists]

The new Faculty was inaugurated and its first Board met on 24 March 1948 with Marston as Dean (Fig 12.13). There is no doubt that, without the Faculty, anaesthesia would not have been recognised as a specialty and anaesthetists would have remained medical officers (as opposed to consultants) indefinitely.

Marston and his Vice-Dean, Bernard Johnson, were a strong team. Marston was affable and adept at persuading others to his point of view. Johnson was thoughtful, innovative, business-like, not always popular, but with a reputation for getting things done and motivating others. The Board, 20 men and one woman, carried their responsibility with great success. From the first, they showed their independent spirit: they insisted on nominating the person who would serve on Council; they ignored the suggestion by the College that they should reduce costs by cutting down on committees, let alone limiting them to Londoners; and they ignored the British Medical Association when it enquired as to the functions of this Faculty.

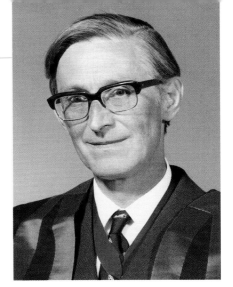

12.14

12.14 Professor Sir James Gordon Robson

Professor of anaesthetics at the Royal Postgraduate Medical School, Hammersmith, the first non-surgeon to be elected Vice-President of the College (1977–79). He was previously Dean of the Faculty of Anaesthetists (1973–76).

The new Faculty adopted many of the practices of the College. Its first scientific meeting, entirely on basic science topics, attracted no fewer than 350 attendees. The first two-part Fellowship was held in November 1953. In the Primary, 65 candidates sat and 9 passed; in the Final, 52 sat and 16 passed.

Founding the Research Department of Anaesthetics jointly with the College proved one of the Faculty's most important initiatives; it has had a great impact both on research activities and on training anaesthetists for academic careers. Later, the British Oxygen Company generously endowed a Chair for the Department. The first Professor, Ronald Woolmer, started basic science courses at a time when such instruction was non-existent. Woolmer liked to end with a 'a good report'; he took students onto the roof of the College and demonstrated loudly and clearly the explosive qualities of cyclopropane to the astonishment of the public in Lincoln's Inn Fields and the lawyers next door!

The Faculty's autonomy within the College and in the wider medical field increased steadily. By the end of 1970, it had representation on every national body on which the College itself was represented. In 1972, Council stated that it considered the Faculty to have 'achieved parity of status and respect with surgery', increased Faculty membership on Council to three and agreed that they should be eligible for election to the office of President. This was a momentous and generous decision, and Council's goodwill was further demonstrated when it elected at the earliest opportunity an anaesthetist to the Vice-Presidency (Sir Gordon Robson, Fig 12.14).

12.15 Inauguration of the College of Anaesthetists of The Royal College of Surgeons, 19 October 1988

Sir Ian Todd, President of The Royal College of Surgeons, sounds the College gong. Standing behind him (left to right) are Michael Rosen (President of the College of Anaesthetists) and some of the past Deans of the Faculty of Anaesthetists, William Woolf Mushin, Aileen Kirkpatrick Adams, Cyril Frederick Scurr, John Francis Nunn, Sir Gordon Robson and John Edmund Riding.

By the 1970s, independent colleges had been established by the pathologists, radiologists, psychiatrists and general practitioners, and many anaesthetists believed the time had come to do the same. A long period of consultation ensued: some anaesthetists argued for complete separation, while others were content with the status quo, which they believed gave them a corporate strength that outweighed the advantages of separation. Yet others sought something in between, such as inclusion of a three-faculty 'Royal College of Surgical Sciences' comprising surgery, dental surgery and anaesthesia, or a title change such as 'Royal College of Surgeons and Anaesthetists'. Council rejected all of these proposals.

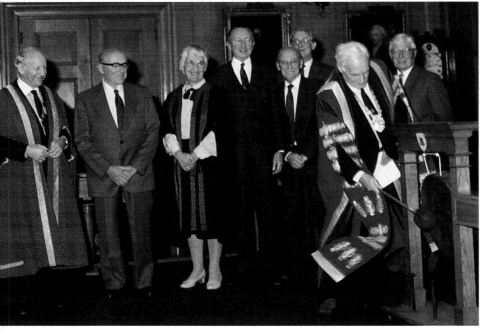

However, in 1986, Council agreed to a new concept, that of 'a College within a College' and put this request to the Privy Council. The formality of changing the Charter went through slowly, but on 19 October 1988 the 'College of Anaesthetists of The Royal College of Surgeons' was inaugurated (Fig 12.15).

Unfortunately, in spite of the initial support for an apparently model compromise that avoided fragmenting the medical profession, protocol defeated it. The Privy Council could not recommend a Royal Charter unless there was constitutional independence; in response, the College of Anaesthetists requested complete separation. The Royal College of Anaesthetists was established on 16 March 1992 and moved to separate premises. The new College was formally opened the following year (Figs 12.16 and 12.17).

12.16 Arms of the College (later Royal College) of Anaesthetists granted 1989

The arms of the new College commemorate its origins by retaining the knotted snakes and the lion's face from the arms of The Royal College of Surgeons of England, while reverting to the blue crenelated cross of the older Company of Surgeons. Blue also indicates that the new College, unlike its parent, includes Scotland. The arms include emblems appropriate to anaesthesia: the opium poppy head and leaves of the coca plant. The supporters are John Snow and Joseph Clover. Its motto is 'It is blessed to relieve pain'.

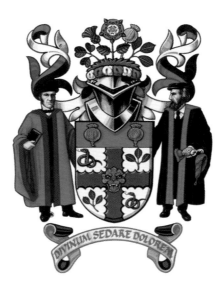
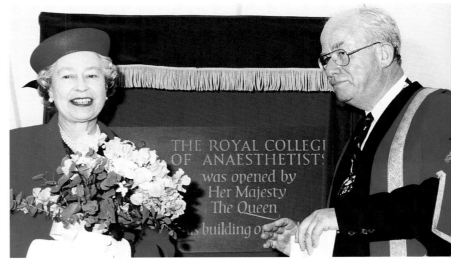

12.17

12.17 HM Queen Elizabeth opens the Royal College of Anaesthetists with the President, Professor Alastair Spence 8 July 1993

[Courtesy Royal College of Anaesthetists]

In forming an academic base for anaesthesia, the Faculty and the Royal College helped to make possible not only great improvements in their own field but to medicine as a whole. Fifty years ago the use of a neuromuscular block demanded meticulous monitoring, and anaesthetists were among the first to instigate clinical measurement and on-line computing for intensive monitoring. Experience in controlling vital functions took anaesthetists out of the operating theatre to treat respiratory problems arising from other causes, and eventually led to the development of the intensive therapy, resuscitation and coronary care that are routine in medicine today.

Audit of anaesthetic-related deaths started as early as the 1950s and evolved into the present National Confidential Enquiry into Peri-operative Deaths (see also Chapter 11).

Developing specialties tend to move into fields where needs are not being met: one of these was relief of pain outside the operating theatre. Both chronic intractable pain and acute post-operative pain are areas in which skills in nerve blocking and familiarity with analgesic drugs have great value. Pain-control teams, often headed by anaesthetists, can now be found in many hospitals and have stimulated fundamental research into pain mechanisms.

The anaesthetist's role today could more accurately be described as that of the peri-operative physician, and perhaps, with the increasing specialisation of medicine, as the only truly general physician still to be found in the hospital service.

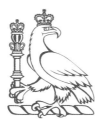

CHAPTER 13

Faculty *of* Dental Surgery

A close relationship existed between dentistry and surgery long before the foundation of the College. Much of John Hunter's practice in the 1760s was in dentistry, as was much of his research, culminating in his classical work on the natural history of the teeth. During the 19th century, a number of College Members practised dentistry, such as George Waite who in 1841 attempted to involve the College in setting standards for dental surgery. Despite unsuccessful initial efforts, the subsequent activity of Sir John Tomes, the pioneer histopathologist (Fig 13.1) and others, brought the Dental Board into being in 1848. Tomes persuaded Council of the need to introduce an examination in dentistry; his efforts culminated in the 1859 Charter, enabling the College to establish a qualifying dental examination. The first examination for the Licentiate of Dental Surgery (LDS) was held in March 1860.

13.1 Sir John Tomes (1815–1895)

Qualifying from the then joint hospitals of Kings and the Middlesex in London, Tomes was house surgeon at the Middlesex, during which time he invented dental forceps accurately adapted to the necks of teeth that replaced the traditional 'key'. He studied the growth of bones and teeth, made histological sections, started a course of lectures in dentistry at the Middlesex, and was a pioneer in the use of ether. 'Tomes began to practice dentistry when it was a trade, and left it a well-equipped profession.' A Fellow of the Royal Society, Tomes was President of the Odonotological Society in 1862 and 1875. He received an Honorary Fellowship of the College in 1883.

By G Meistner

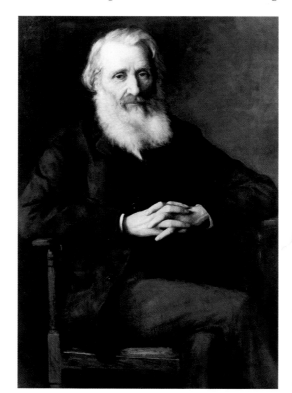

Almost 20 years later the first Register of Dentists was produced as a result of the *Dentist Act* of 1878. The College's influence in undergraduate dental training was dominant throughout this period, and it was not until London and other universities began to establish dental faculties that the influence of the College in undergraduate training diminished. Towards the end of the

1930s, an increasing number of surgical Fellows within the College practised dentistry, in recognition of which the Charter Committee of 1939 suggested revision both in governance and the examination system.

In May 1943, Sir Cuthbert Wallace (Fig 13.2) recommended to Council that permission be sought to institute a higher diploma in dentistry, to be called the Fellowship in Dental Surgery of the Royal College of Surgeons. Despite the difficult times of the Second World War, Council recognised the need to foster the interests of the various surgical specialties, and in July 1944

13.2 Sir Cuthbert Sidney Wallace (1867–1944)

Wallace was educated and began his career as a surgeon in obstetrics at St Thomas's Hospital, where he also served as surgical registrar, senior surgeon and dean of the hospital's medical school. His commitment to the strictest asepsis and his initiatives to modernise and electrify the wards made St Thomas's a source of interest and inspiration to hospital authorities and surgeons around the world. Wallace volunteered for active war service in South Africa and during the First World War, where his economy of time in operating and his defiance of surgical convention won him much renown. In 1915 he successfully treated King George V, who had been thrown from his horse while inspecting troops. At the College Wallace was elected both to the Court and Council. He also served as Vice-President, President, and as a Trustee of the Hunterian Collection. In 1923 and 1929 he was appointed an Examiner in Surgery on the Dental Board.

By A Egerton Cooper

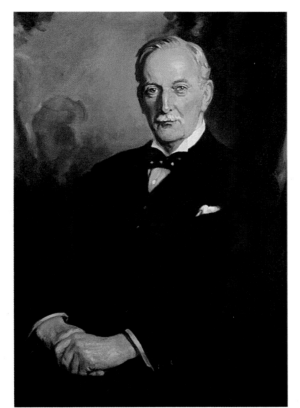

representatives of several specialties – including dental surgery – took up seats on Council. Although the Faculties were not established until 1947, the whole process from their conception by Sir Henry Souttar (see also Fig 15.24) in 1941, to their realisation in less than six years was a remarkable achievement. Under the Presidency of Lord Webb-Johnson (see also Fig 5.6) the College not only encouraged additional surgical specialties in their development, but changed the composition of Council and the tenure of Council members for the first time in almost a century.

The establishment of the Faculty of Dental Surgery was a joint venture between Council and the British Dental Association. Robert Bradlaw (Fig 13.3), a member of the College Board of Examiners for the LDS, proposed to Council the establishment of a joint working party; its recommendations resulted in an application to the Privy Council for a supplemental charter to enable the College to create and regulate faculties. The charter was granted in May 1947 and the Board of the Faculty of Dental Surgery was formally inaugurated on 31 July of that year (Figs 13.4 and 13.5).

To establish a Board of Faculty, Council proposed senior figures for election to the Fellowship in Dental Surgery, choosing names from the London and provincial dental schools, from the armed services, the

13.3 Sir Robert Vivian Bradlaw (1905–1992)

Educated at Cranleigh and Guy's Hospital both as a dental and medical student, Bradlaw spent some time in private practice and as a ship's surgeon. In 1936 he was appointed to the Chair of Dental Surgery in Newcastle-upon-Tyne, where he revolutionised the undergraduate dental curriculum. In 1960 became Dean and Director of Studies at the Institute of Dental Surgery. He also served as Director of the Eastman Dental Hospital and Professor of Oral Medicine at the University of London. Bradlaw helped define the role of dentistry within the new National Health Service and was President of the General Dental Council from 1964 to 1974 as well as the British Dental Association in 1974.

By Rickman

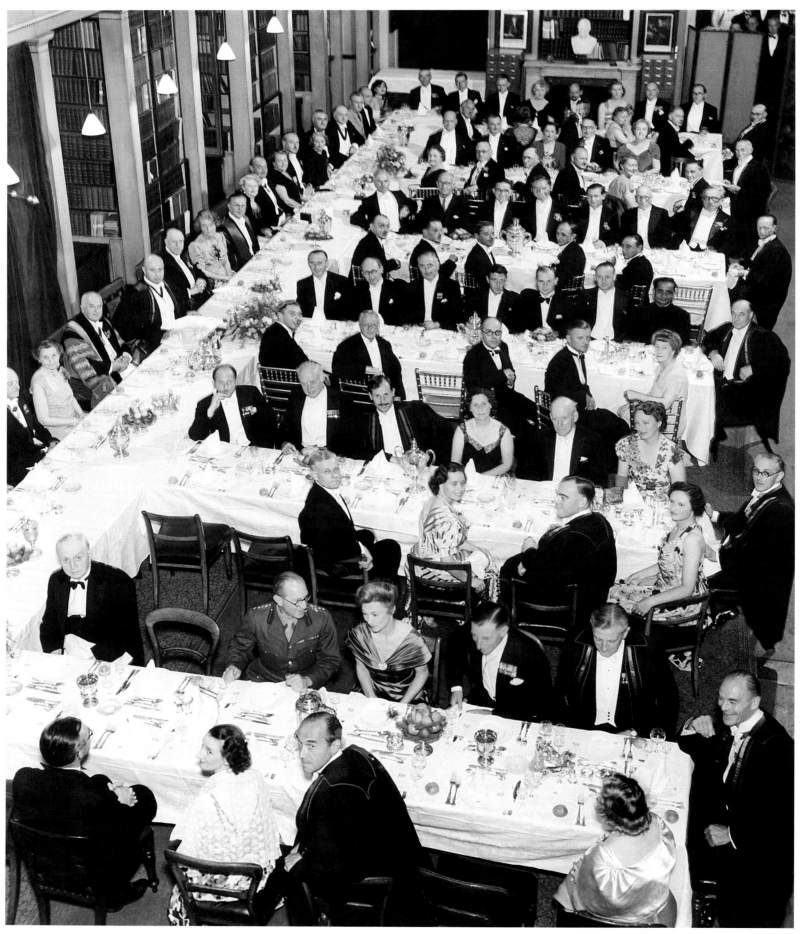

13.4 Second Annual Dinner of the Faculty, 1949

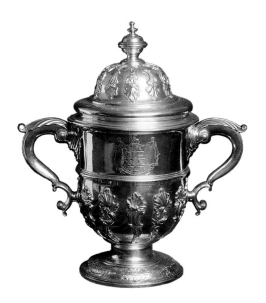

13.5 Pitt Cup

This cup was presented to the College to commemorate the inauguration of the Faculty and Fellowship in Dental Surgery on 31 July 1947. It bears the arms of the Pitt family and was made by John Jacob, London, 1742.

Ministry of Health, the Board of Examination for the LDS, the Dental Board of the UK, the British Dental Association, general practice and the Public Dental Service. As a consequence, the inaugural board drew experience from a very wide range of the profession.

Bradlaw served as the first Dean of the Faculty. His association with the College extended over 22 years. Provision was made for the election of 250 dental Fellows over the next three years, and the committee overseeing the election ensured that the distinguished membership of the Board was upheld.

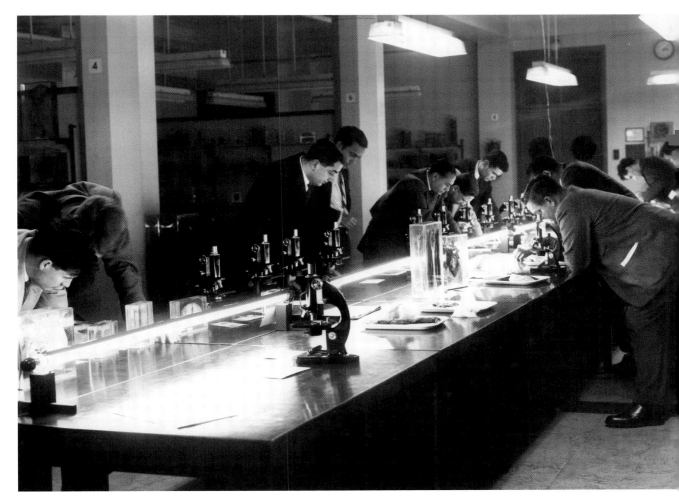

13.6 Students in a dental pathology class in the 1950s

The establishment of the Faculty of Dental Surgery coincided with the establishment of the National Health Service, and its presence ensured parity for consultants in the dental specialties with their counterparts in medicine and surgery.

The Faculty began with two main tasks: first, to establish a programme of education within the College (Fig 13.6) leading to a Fellowship in Dental Surgery by examination and, secondly, to influence the new National Health Service to recognise the part played by dentistry in the delivery of healthcare. Sir William Kelsey Fry (Fig 13.7) helped set up training programmes and develop a Fellowship examination with standards comparable to the surgical examination of the College.

13.7 Sir William Kelsey Fry (1889–1963)

Working with Sir Harold Gillies at Sidcup, he helped pioneer the development of maxillofacial surgery. After the war, he was appointed to the staff at Guy's where he was an outstanding clinician and teacher. During the Second War, he worked at East Grinstead, making it the foremost postgraduate teaching centre. He was largely responsible for the establishment of a postgraduate dental school at the Eastman Dental Hospital, where he lectured in oral surgery. He served as Dean of the Faculty of Dental Surgery from 1950 to 1953.

13.8 Sir Eric Wilfred Fish (1894–1974)

A great researcher, as well as clinician and teacher, Fish was a prodigious writer on numerous topics of considerable practical importance, including the histopathology of enamel, dentine and the dental pulp, the surgical pathology of the mouth and in particular infection of the bone, the stabilisation of full dentures, and the formation and treatment of peridontal disease. He was elected Chairman of the Dental Board of the United Kingdom in 1944 and when it was succeeded by the General Dental Council, became its President. He was Dean of the Faculty in 1958 and was the first Director of the Department of Dental Science.

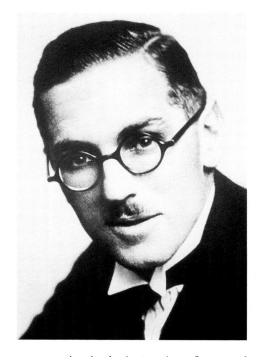

The Fellowship examination, originally proposed in 1939, was finally established in April 1948. It rapidly became the recognised qualification for those seeking senior posts within the National Health Service and universities. In due course it was emulated by the surgical Colleges in Dublin, Edinburgh and Glasgow. The Fellowship of Dental Surgery also had a marked influence overseas, and many dental surgeons from across the world came to study for this award in the Nuffield College and the Institute of Basic Medical Sciences.

The Faculty was responsible for the application of basic scientific knowledge to dentistry and for co-operating in the instruction of postgraduate dental students. Sir Wilfred Fish (Fig 13.8) was appointed as first Director and, with the help of a generous gift from the Leverhulme Trust, developed a successful educational programme. In 1956 Bertram Cohen was appointed as the first Research Fellow in Oral Pathology, and was later appointed to the new Nuffield Research Chair in Dental Science (Fig 13.9).

The Faculty made valuable use of the Buckston Browne Farm at Downe, where David Poswillo established the Chair in Teratology. Professor Newell Johnson succeeded Cohen in the Nuffield Research Chair in 1993. With the closure of the Buckston Browne Farm and the Hunterian Institute, the Department of Dental Science moved to King's College Hospital.

The Fellowship Examination

When the Fellowship in Dental Surgery was introduced, it was the highest dental diploma the College awarded. However, like the FRCS, it changed significantly over the years. In 1948 the Fellowship was a postgraduate examination taken shortly before the end of specialist training,

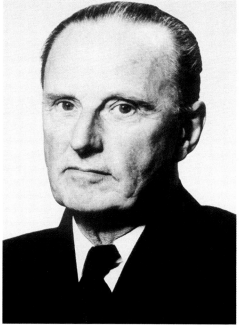

13.8

serving as a measure of suitability for a consultant appointment. With the passing years, the examination was taken earlier in a surgeon's career until it became an essential requirement for entry into higher training: the trainee was no longer assessed on the completion of training. A move to transfer the examination again to the end of the final year of specialist registrar

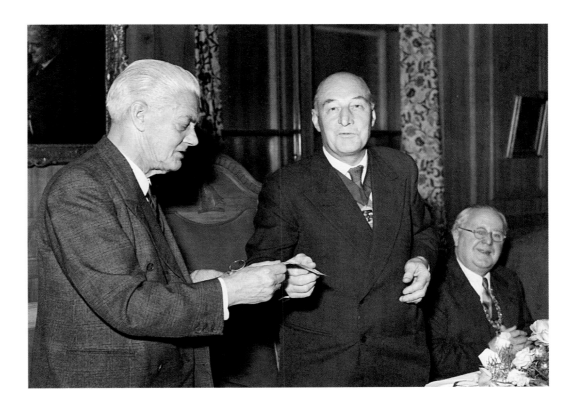

13.9 Lord Nuffield giving a cheque for £100,000 to the Dean of the Faculty of Dental Surgery (Professor F C Wilkinson) to establish a Chair of Dental Research in 1956 (Sir Harry Platt on right)

training was achieved on an intercollegiate basis in 1995, making the Fellowship in Dental Surgery once again a certificate of completion of training, as with the other surgical specialties.

In dentistry, as in surgery, the Primary Fellowship examination gradually became obsolete and was replaced by a new intercollegiate Membership examination as the entry requirement for training in any of the dental specialties. Specialty assessments in an Intercollegiate Fellowship examination ensure that trainees in specialist aspects of dentistry are examined to the highest level at the end of their training time. This has been driven both by educational requirements and the influence of Europe, with the need to harmonise and shorten training. Other diplomas offered alongside the Fellowship help to support the comprehensive educational programme within the Faculty. In addition, Honorary Fellowships are awarded to those who have been outstanding in dental surgery or of single service to the Faculty (Fig 13.10).

Sub-specialisation

In its early days, the Faculty recognised the need for sub-specialty training within dentistry for those not necessarily aspiring to Fellowship status. The initial diploma in orthodontics of 1954 was replaced by the Membership in Orthodontics in 1986; the Diploma in Dental Public Health, instituted in 1965, was replaced by a Membership in Clinical Community Dentistry in 1988. Thanks to Brian Mouatt, Chief Dental Officer, and the General Dental Council, the Board moved with the Dental Faculties of other surgical Colleges to establish Membership examinations in the other sub-specialties of dentistry. The Fellowship and Membership examinations in dentistry are truly intercollegiate ventures, whereas specialist Memberships have made limited progress towards becoming fully intercollegiate.

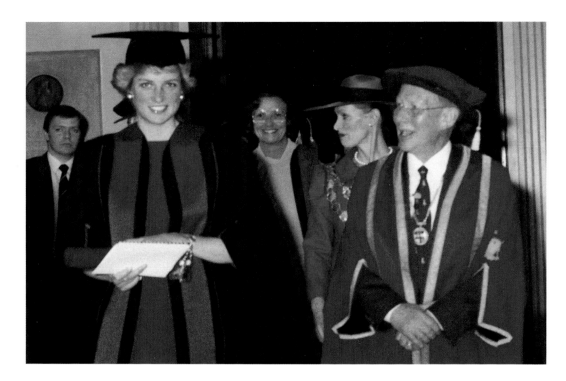

13.10 Her Royal Highness The Princess of Wales being made an Honorary Fellow, 1988, with Professor Gordon Seward, Dean of the Faculty of Dental Surgeons

Education

The need to harmonise education and training for better freedom of movement of individuals throughout the European community profoundly influenced dentistry. The Board of Faculty has been directly involved with many of these changes, in conjunction with the Department of Health and the General Dental Council. When the General Dental Council was established as the sole competent authority for dentistry, an even closer working relationship evolved between all parties under the Specialist Training Advisory Committee. To satisfy European criteria, the curricula of the new Fellowship, Membership and Specialty examinations were revised.

From its inception the Faculty has been involved in education overseas. Surgeons from around the world have taken the Fellowship, and in recent years the Primary Fellowship has been held in many of the countries from which these diplomates were originally drawn. When these countries developed their own Fellowship examinations with equivalent standards, they were granted reciprocity with the College examinations.

The advent of modern technology and the changing structure of the Faculty examination necessitated the development of a distance learning programme to continue its influence overseas, following the lead of the Raven Department of Education for the new MRCS examination with its *STEP* learning programme (Fig 13.11).

No longer is education confined to pre-consultant training: there is now a demand for life-long learning through continuing professional development. The Faculty participates with the rest of the College in the current educational programmes. Dental masterclasses are being developed within the Raven Department of Education Department to meet the needs of specialists.

Relationships with Other Bodies

The committee structure of the Faculty mirrors that of the College, with chairmen serving on the respective College Boards. The Audit Committee is connected to the dental specialty associations, sharing responsibility for the development of guidelines in the sub-specialties of dentistry, which is in turn linked to the overall continuing medical education of the Academy of Medical Royal Colleges.

The Hospital Recognition Committee inspects all senior house officer posts, many recognised jointly for the FRCS Examination for those aspiring to a career in oral and maxillofacial surgery. The Joint Committee for Higher Training in Dentistry is made up of a series of specialist advisory committees for each dental specialty.

A series of specialist advisers maintains the Faculty's regional influence, and ties are being developed with European colleagues and with the establishment of the Union of European Monospecialties. Oral and maxillofacial surgery is an established European specialty under the medical directives, and provides a model for the evolution of other dental specialties, particularly orthodontics.

The Dean has a key role not only within the College but also with external regulatory and advisory bodies, and he was a founder member of the Conference of Medical Royal Colleges, the forerunner of the Academy. As a full member of the Academy of Medical Royal Colleges, the Dean serves on the Joint Consultants Committee. This link between the Faculty and the Department of Health facilitates discussion of all aspects of professional activity, other than those related to terms and conditions of service.

13.11 **St John Crean conducting a seminar on an MFDS Study Day at the College**

The Faculty's seat on the General Dental Council is traditionally filled by the Dean, who also serves on the Specialist Training Advisory Committee. The Dean has similar responsibilities to those of the President of the College and has an equal opportunity to serve as chairman or vice-chairman of the appropriate bodies, ensuring that the Faculty stays at the forefront of discussions over quality of care within the National Health Service.

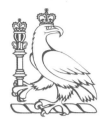

Faculty *of* General Dental Practitioners

C oncern about the place of the general dental practitioner within the Faculty of Dental Surgery came to a head in 1973, when a working party was set up to consider the creation of a membership in general dental practice. The Fellowship of Dental Surgery identified dental surgeons who had completed higher training, and went on to define and introduce training pathways for individual dental specialties. This occurred at a time when initiatives in medicine eventually led to the establishment of the Royal College of General Practitioners, but it took another decade before there was a comparable move in general dental practice. The lack of markers of achievement or any structured training programme made it difficult for generalists to advance their skills. In 1977, work began on the syllabus and regulations for the Membership in General Dental Surgery. The first examination in 1979 served as a model soon adopted by the Scottish and Irish Colleges.

In 1981 the Faculty established a Committee on General Dental Surgery, which became the Advisory Board in General Dental Practice in 1986. In March 1991, Derek Seel (Dean of the Fellowship of Dental Surgery) and Stephen Rear (Chairman of the Advisory Board) approached Council and received the answer that 'Council supports the principle of a Faculty of General Dental Practitioners within The Royal College of Surgeons of England.'

The development of vocational training schemes did much to confirm that general dental practice was a discipline with its own skills and attributes (Fig 14.1). Mandatory vocational training meant that substantial numbers of practitioners in all parts of the United Kingdom were now involved as trainers, trainees, scheme organisers or presenters on the study day course. The Advisers Conference, leaders of the vocational training movement, saw the merits

14.1 Dental practitioners at work

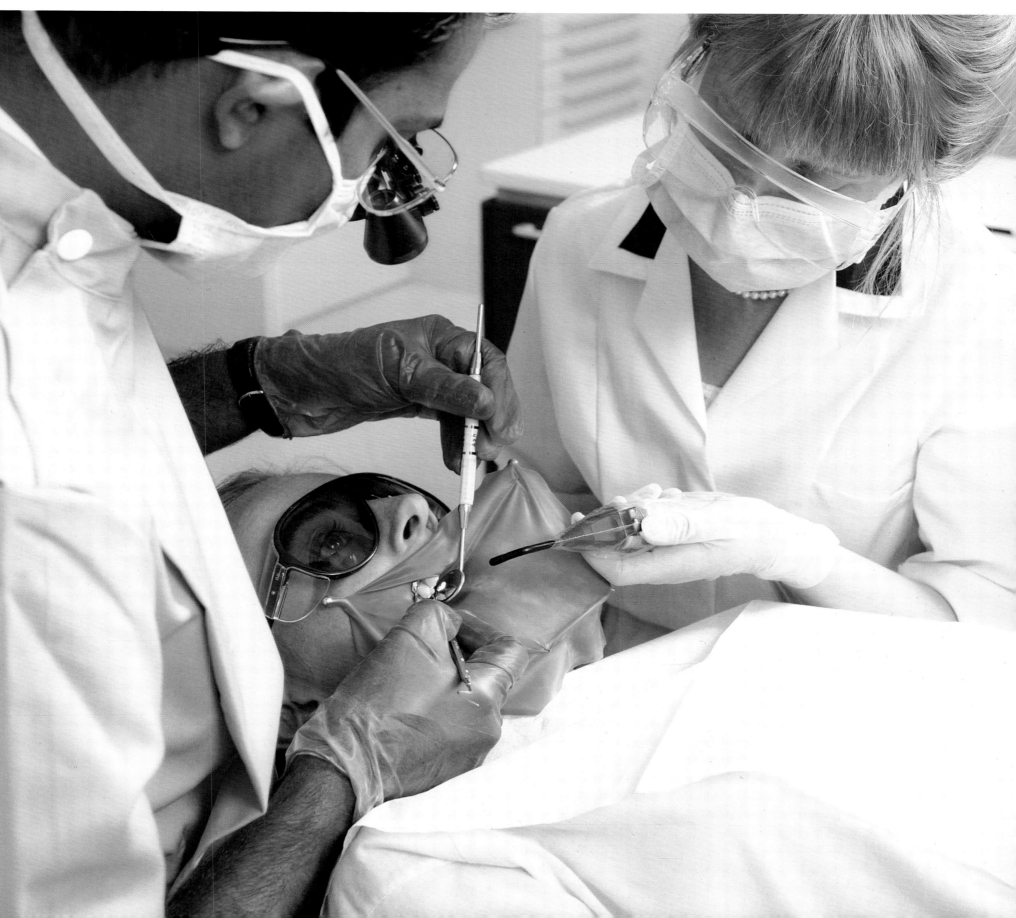

of an academic home for general dental practice and registered a body known as The College of General Dental Practitioners of the United Kingdom, chaired by Peter Lowndes with Malcolm Pendlebury as Secretary.

After a series of meetings starting in May 1991 on the 'neutral ground' of the British Postgraduate Medical Federation, foundation members of the College of General Dental Practitioners and representatives of the Advisory Board reached an accord: the news was well received at the open forum of the British Dental Association conference in Manchester in July, and in October 1991 the College Council reaffirmed its support for a Faculty of General Dental Practitioners (UK) of The Royal College of Surgeons of England. The title and the reference to the United Kingdom resulted from consultations across the whole country, which had produced a strong consensus that general dental practice required a single academic home and that the quadripartite college system of the other specialist faculties should not be replicated.

14.2 FGDP publications promoting quality in general dental practice

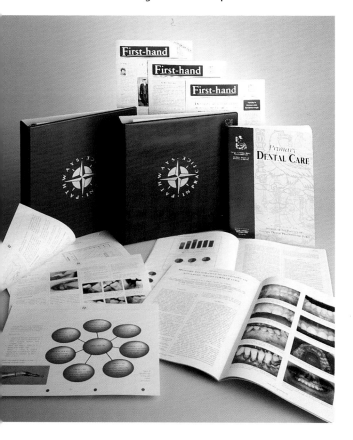

The Faculty Board first met on 16 May 1992 and took on the challenges of finding accommodation in the College, creating a working structure, developing geographic units throughout the UK, attracting members, and establishing a training system and qualification to meet the needs of general dental practice.

The Faculty recruited Anthea Stevens as its first Secretary (later retitled Registrar) and set up committees in education, examinations, finance, membership and research. Their chairmen formed the Dean's Committee for day-to-day management. The Deans of the new Faculty have included Stephen Rear (1992–94), Peter Lowndes (1994–97) and Malcolm Pendlebury (1997–2000). When accommodation on the ground floor of Nuffield College proved too small, the office moved to the fifth floor of the main College building.

As one of its first initiatives, the Faculty designed a series of distance learning texts to support candidates for the Diploma in General Dental Practice under the title *Pathways in Practice*, edited by Professor Peter Rothwell. The Faculty also published its own journal, *Primary Dental Care*, edited by Julian Scott and his successor, Ted Renson (Fig 14.2).

A divisional structure was set up to cover the whole of the United Kingdom. Through this structure regional representatives were elected to the Board of Faculty, although a small number of national seats were voted upon by all members.

The Faculty took over responsibility for the existing title of Member of General Dental Surgery and used it as its senior qualification. It foresaw the early establishment of a junior qualification, the Diploma of General Dental Practice, to signify competence at the level expected two years after qualification. A long-term objective was the development of a fellowship in general dental practice.

Unexpectedly, the Faculty received many requests for training programmes outside the UK, thus echoing in many other places the vision of the initial enthusiasts. Courses and Diploma examinations have been provided in Hong Kong, Malaysia and Singapore, and today the Faculty welcomes many overseas members.

14.3 Malcolm Pendlebury, Dean of the Faculty, left, with new Fellows on FGDP Fellowship Day 1998

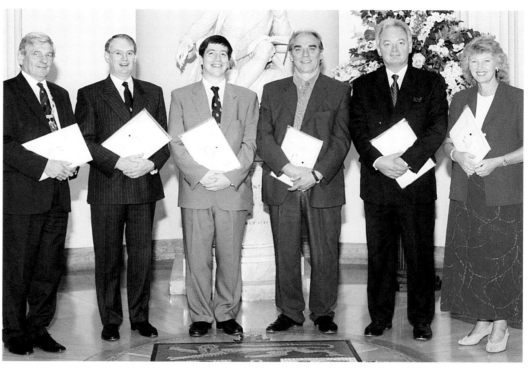

14.3

Recent developments include the establishment of the Fellowship of the Faculty of General Dental Practitioners (Fig 14.3). This Fellowship by assessment marks the ultimate achievement of a mature practitioner. In examinations, reciprocity has been agreed between Part A of the Membership of the Faculty of Dental Surgery and Part I of the Diploma of General Dental Practice, which is now called the Member of the Faculty of General Dental Practitioners.

The Faculty has worked to promote research in primary dental care and has partnerships with a number of institutions, both in the UK and throughout the European Union. It has also formed agreements that will result in structured courses in the clinical disciplines, and has published authoritative statements relating to clinical standards.

After establishing the Faculty and providing it with a working structure, the main challenges were proving its value to the profession and, above all, developing standards of patient care and a career pathway for the profession. The Faculty is now an accepted and essential part of the world of dentistry. It looks to build on this role by promoting standards of training in the interests of improved patient care.

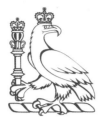

CHAPTER 15

Surgical Specialisation: Emergence *of* the Specialist Associations

The model of the traditional British general surgeon has a long and distinguished pedigree. William Cheselden's innovations in the surgery of cataract were as notable as his contributions to lithotomy, while John Hunter, Percivall Pott and William Blizard were as adept in amputation as they were in dealing with trauma or infection. George Guthrie and Thomas Spencer Wells began their civilian practices in ophthalmology, yet both made significant contributions to abdominal surgery and urology. Jonathan Hutchinson, perhaps the supreme example of the non-specialist, is remembered in a dozen eponyms for his discoveries in dermatology and surgery.

As surgery expanded, surgeons began to concentrate their activities on a specific organ or area of the body, or, in more recent times, on a particular technique such as laparoscopy or microsurgery. This allowed the perfection of specific skills and was followed by surgeons with similar interests meeting to discuss clinical problems and to form specialist associations. These organisations promoted their respective specialties at local, national and international levels and represented the interests of their members, particularly on political and financial matters and surgical areas of controversy. They set standards, laid down the requirements for training programmes and individuals, and identified and certified training units. They usually published a specialist journal.

War was an effective school for surgical specialisation. Expertise acquired in the First World War in the management of fractures, head injuries and burns laid the foundation for the subsequent development of the specialities of orthopaedics, neurosurgery and plastic surgery. These specialties were reinforced during the Second World War. The establishment of the

National Health Service in 1948 led to the provision of specialist services, which had previously been managed by the voluntary hospital system.

Today's 20 or more specialist associations evolved out of the eight for which the College provides regional advisers, and now belong to the Federation of Surgical Specialist Associations.
The College encouraged these developments and has offered accommodation to all associations within the Federation (the majority are currently housed in Lincoln's Inn Fields). Each specialty is represented on Council by invited representatives who are free to take part in all debates. They have relatively short terms in office – usually three years – to ensure that they are au fait with the views of their association.

The Association of Surgeons of Great Britain and Ireland (ASGBI)

ASGBI (Fig 15.1) was founded in 1920 by a group of leading surgeons of the day. The guiding spirit behind the concept was Berkeley Moynihan (Fig 15.2), who had been struck by the lack of cohesion among surgeons as early as 1909. He wrote,

> ...surgeons in one town knew little or nothing of surgeons elsewhere. A surgeon from
> Manchester had never visited an operation theatre in Leeds, nor had ever been asked in

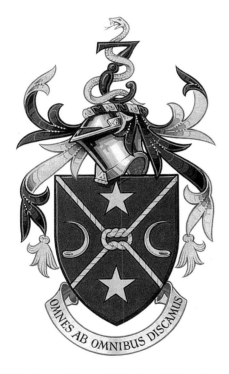

15.1 Coat of Arms of the Association of Surgeons of Great Britain and Ireland

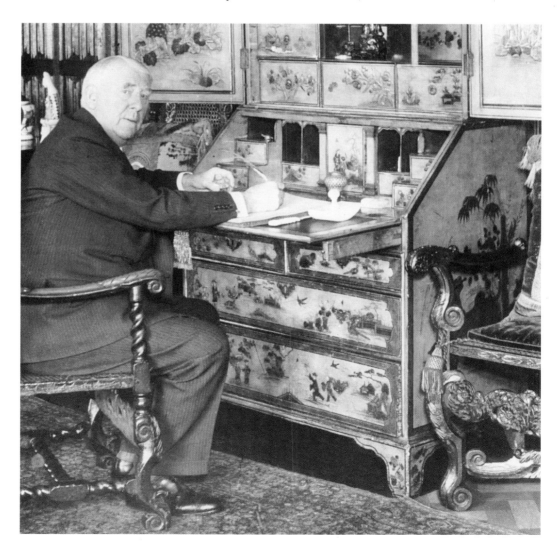

15.2 Lord Moynihan seated at the Chinese Chippendale desk, now in the President's office, that was purchased from his estate and then donated to the College in 1968 by Sir George Martin

Biographical notes for Lord Moynihan accompany Fig 4.22

consultation. As a consequence it was not infrequent to have to listen to disparagement of one surgeon by another; and jealousies, openly expressed, were too often heard.

The founding objectives of the association, therefore, were twofold: advancement of the science and art of surgery, and the promotion of friendship among surgeons.

The first meeting was held in London under the Presidency of Sir John Bland-Sutton (Fig 15.3), the second in Edinburgh, and the third in Leeds under the Presidency of Moynihan himself. Since then meetings have been held in many other centres in England, Scotland, Wales and Ireland. A second annual overseas meeting was initiated in 1985.

Initially, the Fellowship was limited to 250 consultants. Women were first admitted in 1936 and, in 1953, an Associate Fellowship was introduced for a limited number of trainee surgeons.

15.3 Sir John Bland-Sutton (1855–1936)

Bland-Sutton entered Middlesex Hospital as a medical student and subsequently became prosector of anatomy, junior demonstrator, senior demonstrator, lecturer from 1886 to 1896, and consulting surgeon; he was a generous supporter of the hospital as well as curator of its pathology museum. He was a skilled abdominal surgeon. Elected to Council in 1910, Bland-Sutton served as President from 1923 to 1925, was President of the Association of Surgeons and President of the Royal Society of Medicine in 1929. During the war, he collected specimens of gunshot wounds; these were displayed in the College museum but were destroyed in the bombing of 1941.

By John Collier

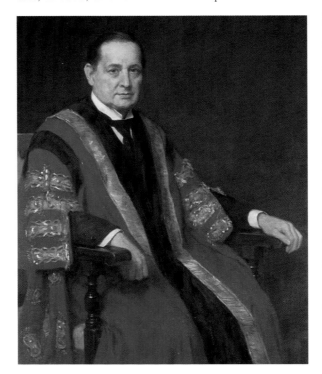

In 1970, 50 years after its foundation, the Fellowship was opened to all consultant surgeons. Currently all specialist registrars are eligible for Affiliate Fellowship and staff grade surgeons for the title of Associate Fellow. Today, the Association is recognised as the specialtist association in general surgery by the government as well as by the profession. It has some 2,000 members.

The Association has encouraged the growth of associations in sub-specialties, inviting them to sit on their council and providing them with a home and secretarial support. Today these include coloproctologists, endoscopic surgeons, upper gastrointestinal surgeons, endocrine surgeons, and vascular surgeons. The Association also has links with the BASO Breast Specialty Group, the British Transplantation Society and the Surgical Research Society. Representatives of the Association of Surgeons in Training and the European Union of Medical Specialties are invited as observers at ASGBI Council meetings.

The Association sponsors a number of prizes. The Moynihan Prize is awarded to the author of the best short paper on new work presented at the annual meeting. The Moynihan Travelling Fellowship enables young surgeons to broaden their surgical education by visiting clinics at home and abroad.

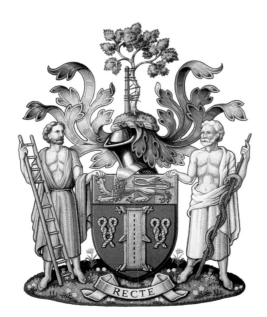

15.4 Coat of Arms of the British Orthopaedic Association

15.5 Sir Harry Platt (1886–1986)

Platt received his orthopaedic training at the Royal National Orthopaedic Hospital in London, the Massachusetts General Hospital and the Children's Hospital in Boston. He returned to Manchester just before the First World War and during the war was surgeon-in-charge of a military orthopaedic hospital there, acquiring considerable experience of nerve injuries and bone grafting. During the Second World War, he was consultant adviser in orthopaedic surgery to the Emergency Medical Service. He was elected to Council in 1940, was Vice-President 1949-1950 and President 1954-1957. He was a founder member of the British Orthopaedic Association and President 1934-1935, as well as a founder member of the Association of Surgeons of Great Britain and Ireland.

By Sir William Hutchinson

The Association's publication, the *British Journal of Surgery*, awards a Travelling Fellowship to a surgeon from overseas to visit and report on surgical practice within the UK. The journal was founded in 1913 by Ernest Hey Groves and Moynihan. During the First World War it published guidelines on the management of war wounds.

The British Orthopaedic Association (BOA)

The British Orthopaedic Association (Fig 15.4) was founded in 1917 after a dinner at the Café Royal in London. At the first meeting of the 20 founder members in 1918, E Muirhead Little became its President. He was succeeded by Robert Jones (see also Fig 4.19), who held the post for six years.

The leaders of orthopaedics at the end of the Second World War – Sir Harry Platt (Fig 15.5), Sir Reginald Watson-Jones (see also Fig 6.12), Sir Henry Osmond-Clarke (Fig 15.6), Norman Capener (Fig 15.7) and Frank Holdsworth (Fig 15.8) – were determined that the lessons learnt by Robert Jones in the building of the Manchester Ship Canal, learnt again in France in 1916, and relearnt in the 1940 Battle of Britain and every theatre of war, should not be forgotten. They wished to make sure that their specialty would never again slide back into general surgery, as it had done between the wars. Existing orthopaedic departments were strengthened at Oswestry and Liverpool; new ones were set up in Birmingham and London.

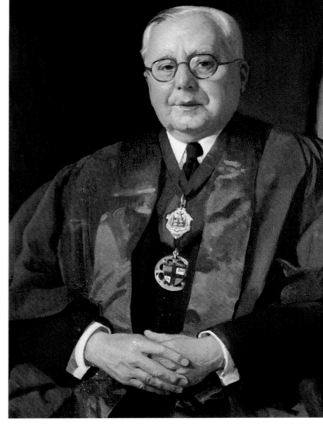

15.5

These developments coincided with the emergence of new alloys to fix bones, and antibiotics to prevent the infection that had hitherto been inseparable from buried foreign material. The concept of replacing worn-out, gliding surfaces of a joint was rapidly developed, from the simple stainless steel cups of Smith Peterson and the acrylic prostheses of Judet, to total joint replacement.

By the time the Association moved into its Lincoln's Inn Fields offices in 1944, membership had grown to 439, of which 375 were practising in the United Kingdom. On its 50th anniversary in 1968, membership was 1,212, with 1,090 based in the UK. At the turn of the 20th century, membership stood at 3,290, of whom 2,750 were UK-based.

15.6 Sir Henry Osmond-Clarke (1905-1986)

Although he held an appointment to the Royal National Orthopaedic Hospital in London, Osmond-Clarke had been trained in Dublin and spent most of his early career in Manchester. His wartime service as consultant in orthopaedic surgery to the Royal Air Force led to many later appointments around the country and involved considerable travel. Osmond-Clarke advised on the development of orthopaedic services as a member of World Health Missions to Israel, India and Persia in the 1950s. His tenure on Council lasted for 16 years, and he was Orthopaedic Surgeon to The Queen from 1965 to 1973. In 1970 he became Vice-President of the College.

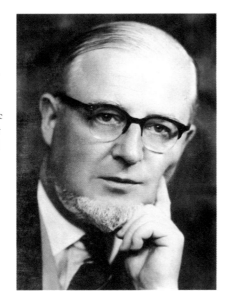

15.7 Norman Leslie Capener (1898–1975)

Capener was responsible for the development of an outstanding regional orthopaedic service in southwest England centred in Exeter that achieved a national and international reputation for its quality of work, teaching and training. His interests were primarily on surgery of the spine and hip, and particularly the treatment of tuberculosis of the spine by lateral rachiotomy. He was President of the British Orthopaedic Association 1958–1960 and on the editorial board of the *Journal of Bone and Joint Surgery* from 1948 to 1966. He was a member of Council from 1961 to 1973, the last three years as Vice-President. His friendship with artist Barbara Hepworth led to her series of surgeons at work. A bronze cast of his hand, also by Barbara Hepworth, was left to the College in his will.

15.8 Sir Frank Wild Holdsworth (1904–1969)

Appointed the first orthopaedic surgeon to the Royal Infirmary, Sheffield in 1937, he was devoted to the practice and teaching of the specialty. He established a paraplegic unit in Sheffield and clinics at Rotherham, Mexborough and Worksop. He was involved in postgraduate training in all specialties in Sheffield and evolved a scheme of rotation of registrar appointments, which was copied throughout the country. He was elected to Council in 1958 and chaired the committee dealing with postgraduate education; at the time of his death he was Vice-President.

15.9 Sir Victor Alexander Haden Horsley (1857–1916)

Horsley combined pathology based on Pasteur with the practice of Lister. Adherence to Lister's methods, along with the use of general anaesthesia and morphia, characterised Horsley's surgery as well as his publicly criticised experiments on animals. His animal experiments, however, led to significant advances in thyroid and pituitary research, and his findings resulted in quarantine and other measures that eventually stamped out rabies and hydrophobia in Britain. His research also focused on the brain and spinal cord, and he took a particular interest in epilepsy. Horsley administered anaesthesia to himself some 50 times at great risk, in order to note the stages of consciousness and the patellar tendon reflex. As an early opponent of tobacco and alcohol for their ill effects on the body, and an avid reformer on a number of other medical issues, he found himself embroiled in numerous political and public debates. From 1882 to 1884 he was Surgical Registrar and he taught pathology, practised and conducted research at University College Hospital from 1884 onwards. Horsley was known for his exceptional skill in exposing the spinal cord.

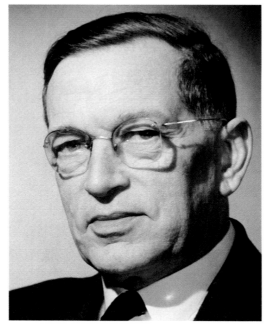

15.7

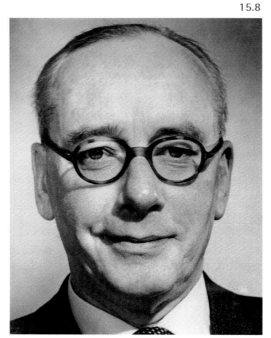

15.8

As orthopaedics split away from general surgery after the First World War, sub-specialisation appeared within orthopaedics after the Second. Hand surgeons were the first to establish their own sub-specialty in 1948. There are now 18 sub-specialist groups under the umbrella of the British Orthopaedic Association Board of Specialist Societies. These groups have memberships ranging from 50 for the surgical oncologist and limb reconstruction surgeons to over 200 for the knee and trauma surgeons.

The Society of British Neurological Surgeons

Neurosurgery was pioneered in the late 19th century by Victor Horsley (Fig 15.9) at the National Hospital for Nervous Diseases at Queen Square; the first meeting of the Society of Neurosurgeons took place there in 1926. The Society of British Neurological Surgeons (Fig 15.10) was created by 17 people attending a dinner meeting at the Athenaeum Club in December 1928. Sir Charles Ballance (Fig 15.11) was elected President and Geoffrey Jefferson Secretary (Fig 15.12). It was the second specialist society to be established, and with the help of Sir Harry Platt, its rules were based on those of the British Orthopaedic Association. It became traditional to hold one of every two annual meetings abroad, a practice that forged powerful links between the society and neurosurgical centres across Europe. Today the Society has about 400 members.

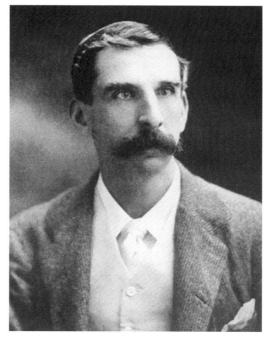

15.9

The technical improvements introduced by Harvey Cushing in Boston had a profound influence on a generation of British neurosurgeons who trained with him, notably Hugh Cairns (see also Fig 5.11) of The London Hospital, who later set up the department in Oxford, Geoffrey Jefferson and Norman Dott in Edinburgh. These early neurosurgeons were aware of the need to be operating neurologists. They made use of the cortical map of Sir David Ferrier, and Sir Charles Sherrington's work at Oxford that won him a Nobel Prize in 1932.

The Second World War expanded the need for neurosurgery both in the armed forces and in civilian practice. The introduction of cerebral angiography in 1927 made it possible to localise brain tumours, and in the 1950s it was the first specialty to benefit from the revolution afforded by computerised tomography. The operating microscope was used from the early 1960s, and stereotactic techniques allowed minimally invasive treatment by ultrasound, lasers and the gamma knife.

15.10

15.10 President's medal of the Society of British Neurological Surgeons

15.11 Sir Charles Alfred Ballance (1856–1936)

In 1888 Ballance took an appointment as aural surgeon at St Thomas's Hospital, and during his tenure significantly improved the department's efficiency and scientific practices. He held the post of surgeon there from 1900 to 1919, and from 1912 to 1926 Ballance was also chief surgeon to the Metropolitan Police. Ballance's involvement with the College was long and varied: he served 19 years on the Court of Examiners, 16 years on Council, and was Vice-President in 1926. Ballance is remembered for being one of the first English surgeons to re-introduce the Hunterian method of experimentation into surgery.

15.12 Sir Geoffrey Jefferson (1886–1961)

Jefferson started his career as house surgeon and demonstrator in anatomy in Manchester and became professor of neurosurgery when a full neurosurgical department was established there in 1934. As an adviser in neurosurgery to the Ministry of Health, Jefferson travelled all over the country with the Emergency Medical Service. In addition to being elected to a Fellowship of the Royal Society in 1947, he held many lectureships, was President of the Association of Surgeons of Great Britain and Ireland, and in 1949 was President of the neurology section of the Royal Society of Medicine. Jefferson served as Chairman of the Clinical Research Board from 1953 to 1959.

By Gerald Kelly

15.11

15.12

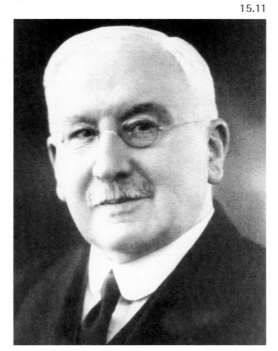

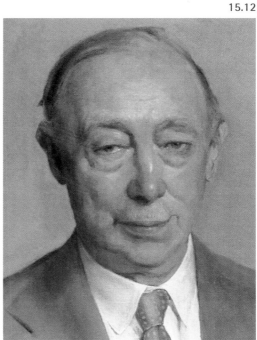

The British Association of Urological Surgeons (BAUS)

Endoscopes for the urinary bladder, stomach and colon had been available from the turn of the century. They changed surgical practice, most notably in urology where transurethral resection of the prostate ultimately led to the branching out of this specialty from general surgery, a development greatly accelerated by new inventions in optics, notably the rod-lens telescope, fibre-light and fibre-optics.

Although the specialty of urology had been well established in three London hospitals (St Peter's, St Paul's and All Saints') as well as in special departments in several hospitals (notably Guy's,

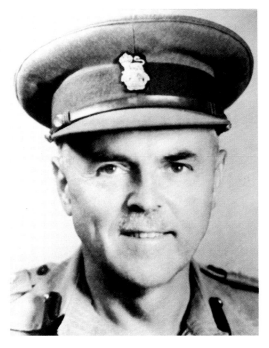

15.13 Ronald Ogier Ward (1886–1971)

After combatant service in the Great War, Ward returned to London and decided to specialise in urology. He was appointed to the St Peter's Hospital for Stone and urologist to the Miller and to the Royal Masonic Hospitals. Between the wars, he built a successful practice and became a leader in urological surgery, and was elected President of the Urological Section of the Royal Society of Medicine in 1935. He was the first President of the British Association of Urological Surgeons and Chairman of the Editorial Committee of the *British Journal of Urology*.

King's, Glasgow Royal Infirmary and Newcastle), there was no specialty association before the Second World War. The *British Journal of Urology* was founded in 1929.

In the mid-1940s Ronald Ogier Ward (Fig 15.13) a consultant at St Peter's, became concerned that there was nobody to speak for urology in discussions about the proposed National Health Service. Lord Webb-Johnson (see also Fig 5.6) advised him that, without a specialist association, urology would have no place on the Consultants' Advisory Committee. The first moves to set up this new body began in December 1944, and within three months the inaugural meeting of the British Association of Urological Surgeons (Home and Overseas) was held in the College.

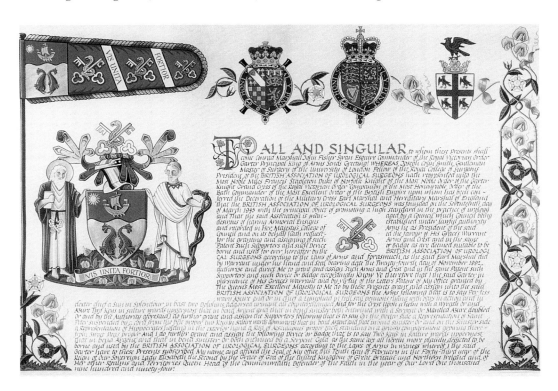

15.14 Charter of the British Association of Urological Surgeons

From the beginning, Webb-Johnson offered the new association a home and secretarial facilities in the College. In 1949, the new association comprised 82 full members from the UK and 55 from overseas; current equivalent figures are 600 and 800, respectively. The cleavage of urology from the main body of general surgery took place relatively slowly. This was primarily due to the general shortage of surgeons; there were simply not enough in the district general hospital to make it possible for one, let alone two, urologists to withdraw from the on-call rota and concentrate on the specialty.

Today the Association (Fig 15.14) has generous new offices in the College building. Its most prestigious awards are the St Peter's and St Paul's Medals. The St Peter's Medal is awarded to 'any subject of the British Isles or Commonwealth who has made a notable contribution to the advancement of urology'. The St Paul's Medal is awarded to 'distinguished colleagues from overseas whose contributions to the Association in particular, or to urology in general, BAUS Council particularly wishes to appreciate and honour'.

The British Association of Otorhinolaryngologists – Head and Neck Surgeons (BAO-HNS)

Founded in 1943, initially as the British Association of Otolaryngologists, BAO-HNS (Fig 15.15) started off with 141 ear, nose and throat surgeons, led by William Mayhew Mollison (President), Lionel Colledge (Vice-President) and Victor Negus (Treasurer), (Fig 15.16). Regional representatives were elected. The consultant adviser in otolaryngology to the Department of Health is a member of its Council, as is the invited member of College Council. The current membership is 1,010.

15.15

The specialty of otorhinolaryngology has its origins in the early 20th century when the otologists (surgeons) joined with the laryngologists (physicians), who also treated diseases of the nose (rhinology) and the chest. Ear-nose-throat became a specialty with a surgical bias, rather than an offshoot of general surgery. Consultant ear, nose and throat surgeons were appointed before the First World War both to teaching hospitals and specialist institutions such as the Hospital for Diseases of the Throat in Golden Square in London. The College recognised the unique nature of the specialty, and Council agreed in May 1947 that there should be an independent Fellowship in Otolaryngology.

The specialty rapidly expanded thanks to the introduction of the microscope to examine the nose, nasopharynx, larynx and pharynx. With antibiotics came an end to acute mastoiditis and its major complications, and fewer operations for tonsils and adenoids. A greater understanding of immunology led to more conservative nasal surgery, and new methods of reconstruction in cases of head and neck cancer have improved function and cosmetic results.

15.16 Sir Victor Ewings Negus (1887–1974)

After service in the First World War, Negus became house surgeon at the Hospital for Diseases of the Throat, Golden Square. He collaborated in the redesign of laryngoscopes, bronchoscopes and oesophagoscopes which were used world-wide, and developed the Negus bronchoscope. After his appointment as a junior surgeon there, he worked most of his career at King's College Hospital. He undertook fundamental research into the comparative anatomy and physiology of the larnyx and paranasal sinuses. He was elected President of the British Association of Otorhinolaryngologists in 1951 and served on Council representing otolaryngology. It was under his Chairmanship of the Hunterian Trustees that the catalogues of the surviving Hunterian specimens were published.

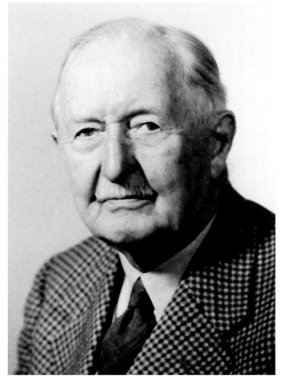

15.16

As with all other specialties, there has been a tendency to sub-specialise. Otology, otoneuro-surgery and skull-based surgery, head and neck surgery, phonosurgery, rhinology, facioplastic surgery and paediatric otorhinolaryngology all have their own society and specialist journal.

15.17 Sir Harold Delf Gillies (1882–1960)

A pioneer in plastic surgery during the First World War at Sidcup Hospital, Gillies continued his practice between the wars on staff at St Bartholomew's and as consultant in plastic surgery to the Royal Navy and the Royal Air Force as well as numerous other hospitals. An excellent teacher, he emphasised the importance of pre-operative planning clinics using exact patterns of flap and pedicle and marking the exact site and length of the incision on the skin. With the outbreak of the Second World War, he organised specialist units throughout the country and ran the largest at Park Prewett Hospital in Basingstoke. He was the founding President of the British Association of Plastic Surgeons and Honorary President of the International Society of Plastic Surgeons.

By Howard Barron

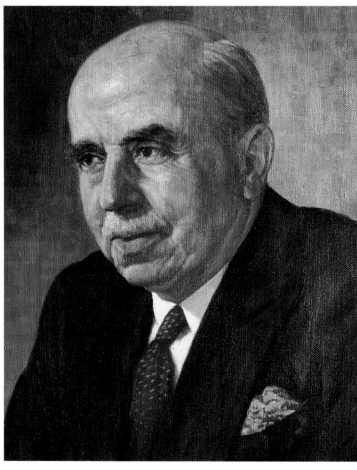

The British Association of Plastic Surgeons (BAPS)

The foundations of British plastic surgery were laid down during the First World War by Sir Harold Gillies (Fig 15.17). Originally an ear, nose and throat surgeon, Gillies appreciated the potential of reconstructive surgery after visiting Val de Grâce Hospital in Paris in 1914. With the backing of Sir William Arbuthnot Lane, he set up the Cambridge Military Hospital, which in 1916 received 2,000 casualties from the Battle of the Somme. Gillies gathered a distinguished team including Henry Tonks, a surgeon-turned-artist and Director of the Slade School who recorded Gillies' surgery in a remarkable series of pastel drawings (Fig 15.18); Sir Ivan Magill (see also Fig 12.9), an anaesthetist who developed a curved endotracheal tube (which not only facilitated faciomaxillary reconstruction but also the development of open chest surgery); and Sir William Kelsey Fry, a surgeon who had trained in dentistry (see also Fig 13.7). Gillies, Thomas Pomfret Kilner, Sir Archibald McIndoe (Fig 15.19) and Rainsford Mowlem made up the 'Big Four' who kept plastic surgery going in the inter-war period.

15.18 Drawing of reconstructive surgery on a soldier during the First World War

By Henry Tonks (1862–1937)

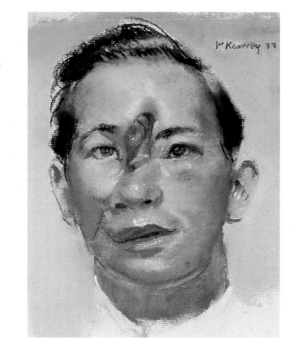

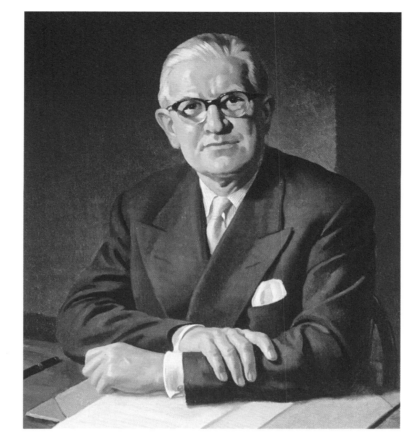

15.19 Sir Archibald Hector McIndoe (1900–1960)

A cousin of Sir Harold Gillies who persuaded him to take up plastic surgery, he is best remembered for his work rehabilitating, both physically and mentally, the badly burned air crew of the RAF. The Guinea Pig Club comprised 600 men who were operated on by McIndoe at East Grinstead. He was elected to Council in 1946 and served as Vice-President in 1958. His most outstanding service to the College was his initiative in raising funds as a member of the finance and appeal committees.

By Edward Halliday

In 1939, war again stimulated the need for reconstructive surgery. The number of plastic surgeons increased tenfold. McIndoe at East Grinstead took over the management of Royal Air Force crews burned in the Battle of Britain who became known as the 'Guinea Pig Club'. Reconstructive principles were applied throughout the body for congenital or acquired deformities. Research into skin grafting stimulated skin cultivation, immunological studies and genetic coding. Tissue transfer searched for reliable donor areas for pedicle and free flaps, and in time microsurgical techniques.

15.20 Coat of Arms of the British Association of Plastic Surgeons

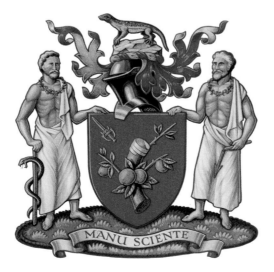

The idea of BAPS (Fig 15.20) started in 1944 but had to be postponed because of the D-Day landings in Normandy. Some 36 surgeons attended the first meeting in November 1946 at the College, when Gillies was elected the first President. The membership is now over 600 from 54 countries. The *British Journal of Plastic Surgery* first appeared in March 1948, and is published monthly.

Within the specialty, sub-specialties have developed, including the British Burn Association, the British Society for Surgery of the Hand, the British Association for Oral and Maxillofacial Surgeons, the British Microsurgical Society and the British Association of Aesthetic Plastic Surgeons.

15.21 George Ernest Gask (1875–1951)

During the First World War, Gask played a distinguished part in the RAMC, securing the most up-to-date treatment for wounds of the chest and lungs, at that time a new specialty. He was particularly concerned with improving the education of younger surgeons and after the war, introduced a full-time professorial unit at Barts. His brilliant team of Sir Thomas Dunhill, Geoffrey Keynes and Ronald Ogier Ward established the success of this innovation. He was active with the *British Journal of Surgery* and succeeded Moynihan as Chairman of the Editorial Committee. He retired from all surgical activity in 1935, but with the outbreak of hostilities in 1939 joined the Radcliffe Infirmary, became involved in the work of the Oxford medical school and became adviser in surgery for the region.

15.22 Arthur Tudor Edwards (1890–1946)

At the Brompton Hospital, Edwards was a pioneer in applying his wartime experience of thoracic surgery to civilian illnesses, including pulmonary tuberculosis, bronchiectasis, tumours of the mediastinum and tumours of the lung. In this work he was supported by his colleagues RA Young, physician, and Ivan Magill, anaesthetist. His work established thoracic surgery as a specialty and himself as its recognised leader. During the Second World War he organised the reception centres for thoracic casualties under the Emergency Medical Service and provided intensive courses of instruction for service thoracic units. He was President of the Society of Thoracic Surgeons and President of the Association for the Study of Diseases of the Chest. He served on Council from 1943 until his early death in 1946.

15.23 Sir Thomas Holmes Sellors (1902–1987)

Following resident medical and surgical appointments at the Middlesex and Brompton Hospitals, Sellors was surgical registrar at the Middlesex. In an era in which tuberculosis was a major bane to society, Sellors' decision to specialise in chest surgery kept him busy: he secured appointments at several London County Council hospitals and sanatoria and started chest units at infirmaries around the country. From the outbreak of the Second World War until his retirement, Sellors worked as an adviser in thoracic surgery at Middlesex, serving also as consultant surgeon to the National Heart Hospital and setting up three new open heart surgery units. Known to a generation of his devoted pupils as 'Uncle Tom', Sellors had a strong dedication to public service, serving on numerous committees and holding many offices, including President of the College from 1969 to 1972.

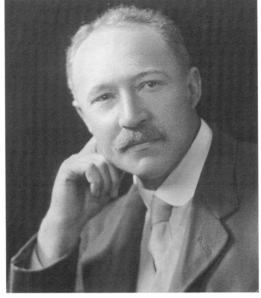
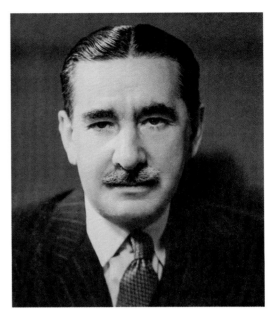

15.21   15.22

The Society of Cardiothoracic Surgeons of Great Britain and Ireland

George Gask (Fig 15.21) had shown in the First World War that for unilateral injuries, the chest could be safely opened and closed. After the war, Arthur Tudor Edwards (Fig 15.22) applied this expertise in civilian practice, first for tuberculosis, and later in tumours, bronchiectasis and diseases of the oesophagus. His work was made possible by the skill of his anaesthetist, Sir Ivan Magill, who had done so much for plastic surgery. Pioneering work went on in the old sanatoria where collapse therapy by phrenic nerve crush, artificial pneumothorax, thoracoplasty and plombage were developed to 'rest the lung'.

Others to develop the new specialty between the wars were Sir Thomas Holmes Sellors (Fig 15.23) and Lord Brock (see also Fig 6.15). Brock had been responsible for fundamental work on the segmental anatomy of the lung to locate lung abscesses; this led to lung resection for segmental disease.

As the threat of tuberculosis receded, thoracic surgeons turned their attention to the heart and the aorta. Mitral valvotomy, which Sir Henry Souttar (Fig 15.24) had shown to be feasible as early as 1925,

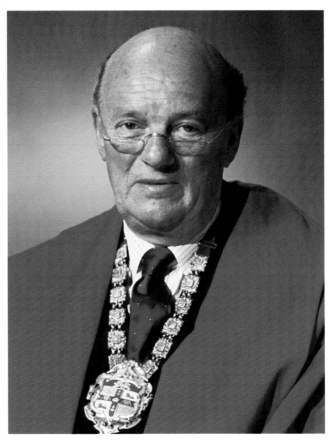

15.23

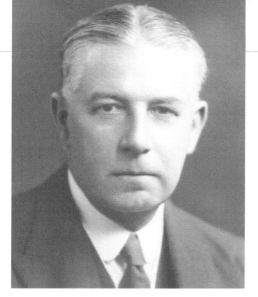

was revived. Holmes Sellors was one of those in the vanguard, confronting the large number of congenital cardiovascular anomalies. Success with patent ductus arteriosus and coarctation of the aorta opened up the field of open-heart surgery with whole-body cooling and circulatory arrest and pump oxygenators in the late 1950s. Bypass of occluded coronary arteries, introduced in 1968, transformed cardiac surgical practice.

15.24 Sir Henry Sessions Souttar (1875–1964)

Souttar enjoyed a great reputation as a teacher, clinician, writer, examiner and as a wise medical politician. He performed an historic operation in 1925 by opening the heart of a 15-year-old girl suffering from mitral stenosis in order to dilate the mitral valve, without using any antibiotic cover or modern means of anaesthesia. It was 22 years before such an operation was repeated. Drawing on his mathematical knowledge and engineering skills, Souttar devised many surgical instruments, such as an atraumatic intestinal needle, an oesophageal tube, a steam cautery and a craniotome. He served on Council from 1933 to 1949 and was Vice-President in 1943–44. Souttar suggested that the College form faculties in anaesthesia and dental surgery, and received Honorary Fellowships from both faculties when founded in 1947 and 1948, respectively.

The first meeting of the Society of Thoracic Surgeons of Great Britain and Ireland took place at the Brompton Hospital in November 1933, under the Presidency of H Moriston Davies and attended by 23 members. The Thoracic Society developed as an offshoot holding its first scientific meeting at the London

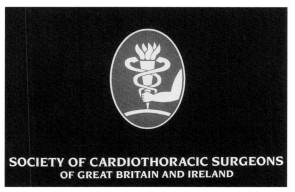

15.25

School of Hygiene and Tropical Medicine in July 1945 and developing its own journal – *Thorax*. The two societies merged again as the Society of Cardiothoracic Surgeons of Great Britain and Ireland in 1984 (Fig 15.25).

The UK Cardiac Surgical Register, the concept of Sir Terence English (Fig 15.26), was established in 1977. It collated post-operative deaths from all UK National Health Service cardiac units,

15.26 Sir Terence English (b. 1932)

Born in South Africa, English came to the UK in 1955 to study medicine at Guy's. He trained under Lord Brock and Donald Ross and then at the Brompton and National Heart Hospitals. Appointed a consultant at Papworth and Addenbrooke's Hospitals, he established the UK Cardiac Surgical Register in 1977 and performed Britain's first successful heart transplant in 1979. He was President of the International Society of Heart Transplantation 1985–86, President of the College 1989–92 and President of the BMA 1995–96. He is currently Master of St Catharine's College, Cambridge.

By David Poole

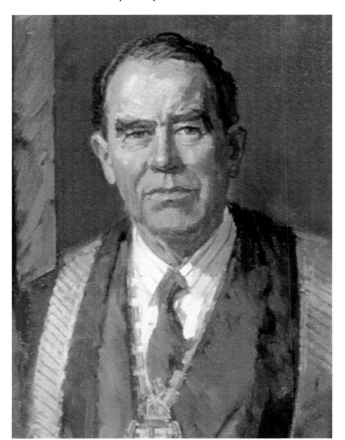

and was the first attempt to collect national activity and outcome data. Cardiac surgery has remained in the spotlight, since failure to achieve the expected outcome can be lethal. A more comprehensive data collection system was introduced in 1994 covering demographic, procedural and outcome information on all patients undergoing cardiac and thoracic surgery. The Cardiothoracic Society has retained its position as the leading specialty in the collection of data and exploring methods of external validation.

The British Association of Paediatric Surgeons

In the 1950s only a handful of surgeons in Great Britain were engaged solely in paediatric practice, the majority of these working in Scotland: many others combined their paediatric interest with adult surgery.

15.27 Sir Denis John Wolko Browne (1892–1967)

Born in Australia, Browne moved to England during the First World War and pursued clinical studies at the Middlesex and London Hospitals. He worked at Queen Mary's Hospital for Children from 1928 to 1957. Browne made numerous contributions to the development of practical methods of treatment of congenital abnormalities, such as devising a simple technique for the repair of cleft palate and hare-lip. He not only had a pioneering role in neonatal surgery, but also advocated looking on the child patient as a whole and considering treatments in relation to the child's growth and development. Browne was Vice-President of the British Medical Association's Section of Child Health in 1952.

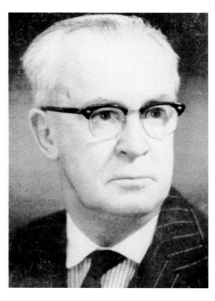

The idea of a paediatric association was fostered by Sir Denis Browne (Fig 15.27), Robert Zachary, David Waterston and Peter Rickman. Most of the 50–60 paediatric surgeons world-wide were approached, and in 1953 the British Association of Paediatric Surgeons (Fig 15.28) was formed, with Browne as its first president.

From its start, the Association was a truly international fellowship, its first meeting being attended by surgeons from Australia, Canada, France, Germany, the Netherlands, Italy, Scandinavia, South Africa and the United States. Annual conferences have toured Europe and the United Kingdom, one of the most successful being held in Jersey. Currently the Association has 920 members, of whom 670 are from overseas, representing 72 countries. Paediatric specialists integrate closely with other specialties including obstetrics, neonatology, paediatrics, oncology and nephrology. In 1965 the Association joined forces with the *Journal of Paediatric Surgery* and a close relationship has existed ever since.

Nowhere is the gap between specialists and generalists more apparent than in paediatrics. The surgical provision for non-specialist procedure is met by general surgeons with a paediatric interest. However, very few higher surgical trainees currently entering the specialist FRCS diploma examination have chosen paediatrics as their sub-specialty; the Association is vigorously engaged in addressing this problem.

15.28

The British Association for Accident and Emergency Medicine

The Association (Fig 15.29) was founded initially in 1967 as the Casualty Surgeons' Association at a time when senior casualty officers had negotiated the establishment of several consultant posts. Since then, the Association has been closely involved with the dramatic improvement in training, in the standards of work and in the organisation of accident and emergency departments. It was also involved in the creation of an Intercollegiate Faculty

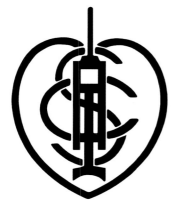

15.29 British Association for Accident and Emergency Medicine

of Accident and Emergency Medicine, inaugurated in 1993, which has conducted its own exit examinations since 1996. The specialty continues to grow and the association has approximately 1,100 members.

The Association of Surgeons in Training (ASIT)

The Association (Fig 15.30) started in 1976 and welcomed trainees from all specialties except orthopaedics (which has its own association). The original membership was limited to senior registrars and lecturers but with the changed structure of training in recent years, this has been broadened. All surgical trainees became eligible for full membership in 1998. Membership in 1976 was 84; today it is approximately 700. The administration of the Association is based in the offices of the ASGBI where the difficult task of tracking the ever-changing trainee population is undertaken.

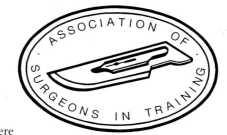

15.30

The Association is represented on most national bodies involved with surgical training and therefore has a powerful influence on surgical governance.

The European Union of Medical Specialists (UEMS)

The aim of the *Treaty of Rome* in 1957 was to produce a peaceful, united Europe without internal barriers, allowing free movement of goods, services, persons and capital across national borders. In order to remove all restrictions on the freedom to provide services, member states were required to recognise one another's qualifying diplomas. This mutual recognition of the general and specialist diplomas was based on a minimum period of education and training, rather than the content of the diploma or the competency of individual surgeons.

The UEMS was created in 1958 to equate standards of specialist medical practice in Europe. In 1993, European boards were founded in each branch of medicine. The European Board of Surgery attaches great importance to the maintenance of a common trunk as part of each specialist training programme. Currently, a European qualification is voluntary; however, the presence of these qualifications establishes a European benchmark of quality control. The European Board of Surgery is also studying the problems of certification of practising surgeons. The establishment of markers of quality is in keeping with the College's own mission of setting and maintaining the highest standards of surgical care for its Fellows and members.

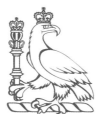

CHAPTER 16

The College Library and Lumley Study Centre: Instruction and Inspiration

T he Library first opened to the public in 1828. Its beginnings were not auspicious. The Company of Barber-Surgeons had collected a library that included surgical books, but when the barbers and surgeons separated in 1745, the ownership of the books was disputed and, in the end, they were sold for £13.

John Hunter deplored this lack of interest in the printed record of surgical knowledge. He wrote to the Company of Surgeons in 1786, urging them to form a new library, saying,

> *Gentlemen:* At this period, in which the surgeons of Great Britain have deservedly acquired the highest reputation in Europe, both by their practice and publications, it appears to be a reflection upon them that the Corporation of Surgeons of London should not be possessed of a public Surgical Library, a circumstance so extraordinary that foreigners can hardly believe it.

> If a custom had been established at the time the surgeons were incorporated that every member should send a copy of his publications to the Company's Library, it would have at present contained the works of many of the best writers in surgery, which might have proved a valuable collection of instructions for the improvement of the profession.

> As the smallest beginnings may in the end lead to the greatest acquisitions I have done myself the honour of presenting to the company through your hands the few observations on Anatomy and Surgery which I have published: and should the other members of that body be induced to follow my example and by presenting their works

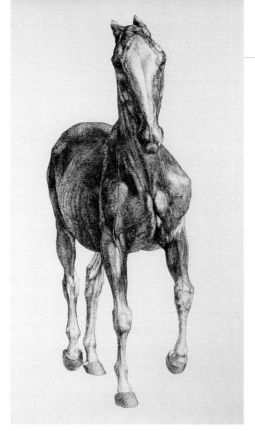

16.1 From *The Anatomy of the Horse,*
published in 1766

By George Stubbs

16.2 William Clift (1775–1849)

John Hunter's amanuensis and assistant, Clift was
an excellent draftsman, and made many original
contributions to osteology and comparative anatomy.
He became a Fellow of the Royal Society in 1823.
After Hunter's death Clift remained in charge of the
collection, and was dismayed when he learned that
Everard Home had burnt many of Hunter's papers.

establish a Library which shall hereafter become both a public benefit and an honour to
the Corporation of Surgeons, I shall consider it as one of the happiest events of my life
to have been at all instrumental in such an establishment.

Hunter's suggestion was not taken up. Consequently, at the Company's re-founding in 1800
as the Royal College of Surgeons in London, it still had no books. When the special committee
of the newly formed College drew up the rules for the care of the Hunterian collection,
it envisaged a library as an integral part of the museum. The Board of Curators that was to
manage the museum began to collect a library. Twelve of the books belonging to Hunter's
estate that had not been scattered at auction were donated by his executors, and books
were bought for the use of Everard Home and William Clift who were working on Hunter's
collections in comparative anatomy.

The first recorded purchases were Stubbs' *The Anatomy of the Horse* (Fig 16.1), Camper's
Description d'un Éléphant, the Annales of the Natural History Museum in Paris, and Shaw's
Naturalist's Miscellany. Serious collecting on a large scale began in 1807 when the Board of
Curators considered the foundation of a library so important that they had 'peculiar gratification
in recording donations of more than 800 volumes'. Generous founding donations were given
by Sir Charles Blicke, a past Master of the College; the widow of William Sharpe, a former
member of Court; Sir Anthony Carlisle, who later became President in 1828 and 1837; and
William Long, the second Master of the College. The historical significance of these donations
cannot be overestimated. To Sharpe and Carlisle the Library owes many 17th century medical
books of great interest, and to Carlisle and Long most of its examples of English Tudor surgery.

In the early years, the work of the Library was carried
out by William Clift, Conservator of the Museum and
John Hunter's last secretary (Fig 16.2). The Court of
the Council appointed the Secretary as Keeper of the
Library, but Clift did the work. Although Hunter's
personal library had by then already been sold, his
manuscripts came to the College along with his
museum. These manuscripts represent a lifetime's
research in surgery and every branch of natural
science as understood in the 18th century. From them

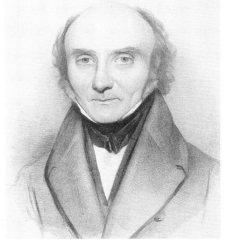

16.2

Clift and Home drew detail and inspiration for their own work. Aside from Hunter's manuscripts,
the Library holds the complete printed record of his work, supplemented by an extraordinary
collection of approximately 1,000 autographed letters gathered by the Hunter and Baillie families
during nearly 200 years of contacts with the most distinguished medical, legal and literary
personalities of their time.

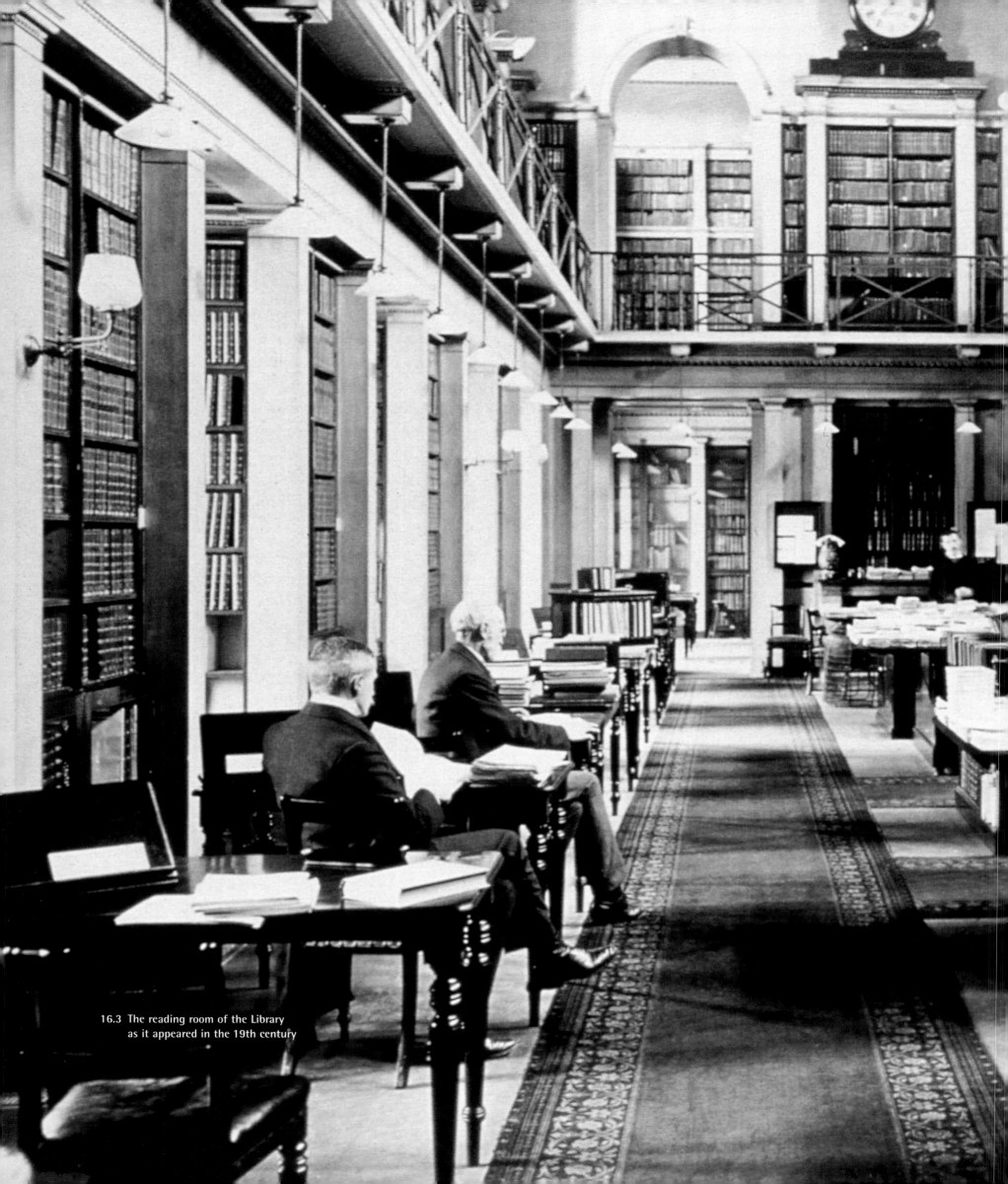

16.3 The reading room of the Library
       as it appeared in the 19th century

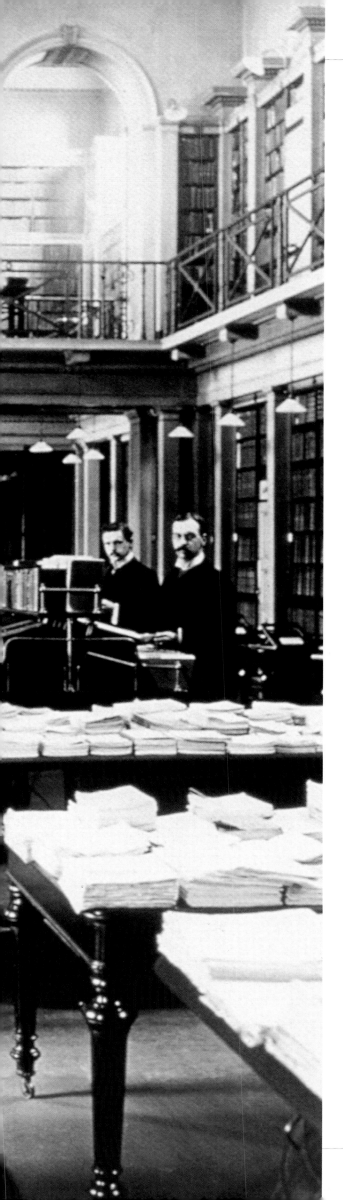

Robert Willis was appointed as first Librarian to the College in 1828, and Richard Owen (see also Fig 3.23) was called in to help Clift in the museum. Between 1834 and 1836, not long after the opening of the Library, the College was rebuilt by Sir Charles Barry. The elegant splendour of the reading room – which was extended in 1887 through the generous benefaction of Sir Erasmus Wilson (see also Fig 3.17) – survives today as a living link with those early years (Fig 16.3). When the College was hit by an incendiary bomb in 1941, it was thanks to the strength of the cast-iron fire doors of the Library that the front of the College survived at all.

Willis carried out his duties with industry and vision until his retirement in 1845. He arranged books in subject groups and not only completed the author catalogues but recast them into a complete classified catalogue, which was printed in 1842. In the middle of the 19th century, the Library was described as follows in Charles Dicken's magazine, *Household Words*:

> The Library is a noble, large room, of excellent proportions, occupying the whole length in front, having tall plate-glass embayed windows, each with its table and chair; and, in each of which, the passers-by in Lincoln's Inn Fields may generally see a live surgeon framed and glazed, busily occupied with his books, or still more busily helping to keep up the tide of gossip for which the place is celebrated. For some twenty feet from the floor on all sides the walls are lined with books. Above this, and just under the handsomely panelled roof, hang portraits of old surgeons, each famous in his time.

Unfortunately, no successor was appointed to Willis. A period of stagnation ensued during which Thomas Stone and John Chatto struggled to keep the Library going. In 1853 Chatto was appointed Librarian, but did not receive any assistance for 34 years; at last, a year before his death at the age of 78, he was given an assistant to help compile a printed catalogue of the Library. That assistant was Charles Hewitt who was to be appointed the first Librarian of the Royal Society of Medicine in 1907.

By April 1887, when Chatto died, the Library collection had doubled to almost 40,000 books, but its arrangement was chaotic. Council realised that it needed a trained librarian and chose James Blake Bailey, who had been trained at the Radcliffe Science Library in Oxford and was then Librarian of the Medico-Chirurgical Society. Hewitt continued as Bailey's assistant and was joined by Arthur Fusedale, who served the College for 50 years. Bailey refashioned the Library within a decade and reorganised it to fit the extra space added by the College, thanks to Wilson's donation. The printed catalogue was discontinued, and Bailey began a card catalogue that is still in use today for all pre-1850 material not yet transferred to computerised records. Bailey pioneered the move to card catalogues at a time when few libraries had them. He then produced a separate list of the periodicals in the Library – the first such list of medical periodicals printed in the country – which demonstrated that the College owned one of the best collections of medical and scientific periodicals in Europe. Chatto had proposed indexing the periodicals, but Bailey pointed out that an effort to index medical periodicals (the forerunner to *Index Medicus*) was already under way in the United States. Bailey also interested himself in the College's fine furniture and clocks and made sure they were in good repair. Sadly, he died at the age of 48 in 1897.

There then followed another period of stagnation, particularly after Hewitt left to join the Royal Society of Medicine in 1907. Victor Plarr, Librarian of King's College, London, succeeded Bailey. According to later College Librarian William LeFanu (Fig 16.4),

> [Victor Plarr] was a sound librarian of the old school, a scholar and a poet, but he lacked
> Bailey's drive, and he joined the College just when a lethargy of false economy was
> settling on it. Keith, [Sir Arthur Keith] who joined it 11 years later, has described it as
> a patriarchal society into which modern methods could with difficulty be introduced.
> Plarr, who was Librarian till 1929, was never allowed a telephone or a typewriter.
> ... Plarr's memorial is in the catalogues which he compiled and in his great record of
> the Lives of the Fellows since 1843, published after his death.

Following Plarr's death in 1929, the Council created the post of Honorary Librarian especially

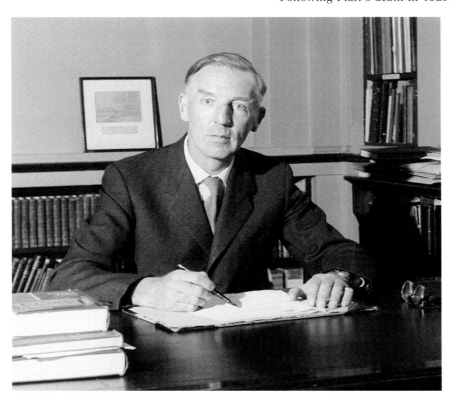

16.4 William LeFanu (1904–1995), Librarian of the College from 1930 to 1968

for Sir D'Arcy Power, a past Vice-President, who was distinguished as both surgeon and historian. A few months later, LeFanu was appointed as assistant to Sir D'Arcy. At last modern methods began to be introduced – a typewriter and telephone were provided, Council made available adequate storage space, and the great collection of periodicals was properly arranged in 1937.

When the Second World War broke out in 1939, the contents of the Library were evacuated to Downton Castle in Shropshire, thereby escaping the bomb that damaged the rest of the College in 1941. The Library was the one great educational asset of the College that survived the Second World War. Unfortunately, the years immediately afterwards were again difficult, as the number of Library staff was reduced and even the typewriter was requisitioned. However, thanks to the efforts of LeFanu, with the support of Sir Geoffrey Keynes (who had succeeded Sir D'Arcy Power as Honorary Librarian) and of Council, the Library was included in the rebuilding and redevelopment of the College in the 1950s and was able to provide a revitalised service to the College.

LeFanu retired in 1968 after a most distinguished career during the course of which he became known internationally in the field of medical librarianship. Eustace Cornelius was then appointed Librarian, having served as LeFanu's assistant since 1948 and helped in the post-war reconstruction. He served as Librarian for 18 years until he retired in 1986, although he continued undaunted thereafter in his work for the *Lives of the Fellows*. Looking back to those immediate post-war years when he first joined the Library, Cornelius can still remember how it was his duty in the winter months to see to the fires that were provided in the reading room and Library office. Samuel Wood, who worked in the Library for a record 70 years, was also a familiar figure. During the 1970s and into the 1980s the Library was heavily used by the staff and resident students of the Institute of Basic Medical Sciences and subsequently the Hunterian Institute.

Medicine in general, and surgery in particular, evolved dramatically after the Second World War. Keeping up with these changes became increasingly difficult, as the number of published journal articles grew exponentially. In 1966, the paper volumes of *Index Medicus* were computerised, and medical librarians all over the world dialed into a database held at the United States' National Library of Medicine in Maryland. Today, the medical profession takes for granted the availability of Medline over the Internet, and electronic versions of journals are commonplace.

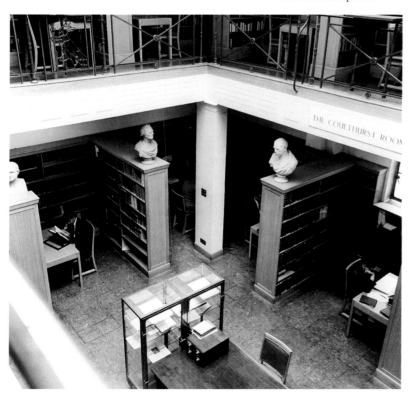

16.5 **The Coulthurst Room**

Ian Lyle, who took over as Librarian when Cornelius retired, shared in those times, having been appointed to the staff in 1966. Lyle served as Librarian until ill-health obliged him to retire in 1997. During his tenure, the Library underwent radical change, including establishment in 1994 of the Heritage Department, which combined the museums and Library under the direction of a Keeper of the College Collections.

Lumley Study Centre

By the late 1980s, the College had already begun to set a course for itself that was to have major consequences for the Library. A working party was set up in 1990–91 to look into Library services after closure of the Hunterian Institute. It was decided to provide a separate study facility for surgeons-in-training, and the Lumley Study Centre was conceived. Hand-in-hand with the development of the Raven Department of Education and the changes in education for surgeons, the educational resources team identified a need for a supporting study centre to contain training materials in a variety of formats. The Coulthurst Room (Fig 16.5) was ideally placed for the proposed Centre, between the Reading Room and the Education Department with direct access from both sides. The purpose of the Centre was to be continuing professional education.

Users were to have access to inter-active multimedia and audio-visual programmes, databases, books and journals.

Council agreed to the proposal, and in December 1994 Richard and Henry Lumley, the chief benefactors, formally opened the Lumley Study Centre. A librarian was appointed that month, supported by one full-time and one shared assistant from the existing staff. The hardware in the multimedia gallery consisted of a small computer network of six IBM-compatible computers, one PowerMac, four video-presenters and a laserdisc player. A small collection of videos was passed on from the Library, and the specialty associations contributed a number of video programmes. The Centre took printed materials published within the previous ten years and gave older books and journals back to the Library.

The main tasks for the staff in the first six months were to develop the collections in the multimedia gallery and to choose library management software for the book catalogue. Heavy emphasis was placed upon the opinions of the users. Strategies were conceived for procuring materials using a standard evaluation process. The idea was to integrate computer materials, produced either commercially or in-house, into existing courses and to make these programmes available to users.

Within three months of its opening, it became clear that the Centre's lower floor needed refurbishment. A generous donation from the Worshipful Company of Barbers funded a new enquiry desk, the lower floor was reshelved, and the Centre was connected to the College's communications network cabling. The staff enquiry point and new layout of printed books and journals had an immediate effect on the number of users, who found it easier to approach staff for help with multimedia programmes and other questions **(Fig 16.6)**.

16.6 **The Lumley Study Centre**

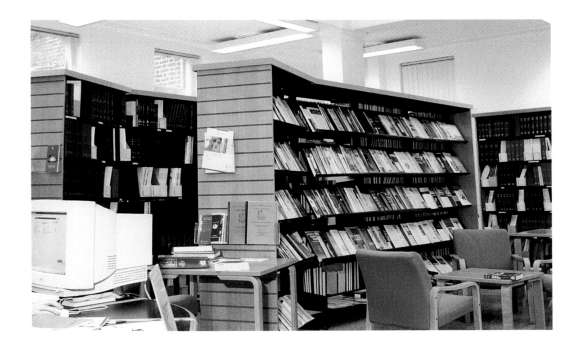

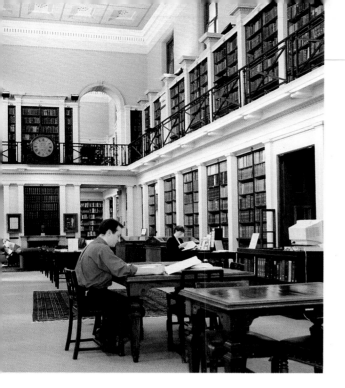

16.7 Modern view of the Reading Room

Keeping Pace with Information Technology

In July 1995, Council agreed to automate the Library catalogue; within three months, the Lumley Study Centre book stock and 6,000 Library titles – 10,000 items in all – had been installed on the Unicorn Library Management system. Use of the Centre expanded, and daily visitors increased over 50 per cent, peaking during the weeks when residential courses were taking place. Internet access became available through some computer terminals in the gallery.

In 1998, three-and-a-half years after the Lumley Study Centre was opened, the College cabling was upgraded, and new computers replaced the old. The installation of web-based software for Unicorn has made it possible for the Library catalogue, distance learning material and medical databases such as Medline and Cochrane to be viewed by Fellows and accredited trainees via the Internet.

As the College celebrates its bicentenary, the Library encompasses a wide variety of services and brings together modern information resources with the archive and historical collections housed within its walls (Fig 16.7). A continuing programme of conservation helps keep the Library's resources in good condition for future users (Fig 16.8). Thalia Knight took office as College Librarian in June 1998 and was charged with reintegration of the Library and Lumley Study Centre services. A five-year development plan was produced with the aim of providing library, archive and information services of the highest professional standards to all its Fellows, Members, trainees, administrative staff of the College and to scholars of surgical history.

16.8 A paper restorer at work on one of the rare books during part of the annual conservation project

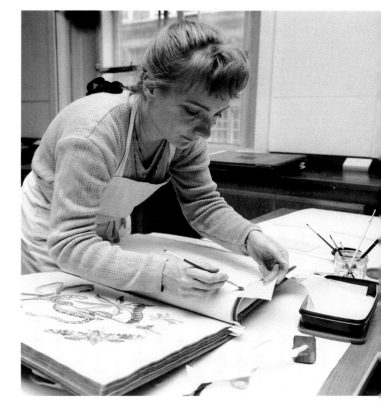

16.8

Users will have access to services and information from their homes and offices via the Internet as well as at the College. The Library will support life-long education and training of surgeons, as well as preserve the record of surgical history. In the words of William LeFanu, it will be 'an enduring memorial of human achievement, from which successive generations can draw instruction and inspiration'.

Treasures in the Library

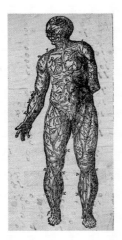

The Englishmans Treasure, with the True Anatomie of Mans Body by **Thomas Vicary (1641 edition)**

John Halle in 1565 wrote of 'the example of good Master Vicarie...who was the first that ever wrote a treatyse of Anatomye in English (to the profite of his breatheren chururgiens and the helpe of yonge students)'. This clearly referred to an earlier edition of Vicary's famous book, which appeared in at least eleven editions between 1577 and 1651. Vicary is thought to have been born sometime between 1490 and 1500. He was the reigning Master who, in 1540, received from King Henry VIII the Charter of Incorporation of the Company of Barber Surgeons. The manuscript for this book (which contains, as so many did, plagiarisms of an earlier anatomical work) was probably found among his papers and published after his death.

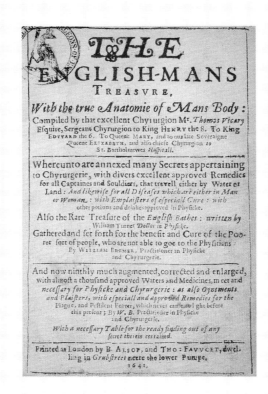

From the *Feldtbuch der Wundartzney* by Hans von Gersdorff (c. 1480–1540); published in Strasbourg, 1535

This lovely woodcut of a 'wound man' is typical of figures that appear in several medieval anatomy books to illustrate various blows and lacerations to the human body by weapons such as clubs and knives. The first edition of the *Feldtbuch* appeared in 1517. The book's many illustrations are valuable for depicting not only surgical practices of the day but also aspects of social history, such as costumes and the interiors of houses. Of particular interest are the comical advertising jingles found throughout the book, for example:

> When I've been hit in hip or thigh
> and wounded so that death is nigh
> I hope that God will stand by me
> and grant me Gersdorff's surgery

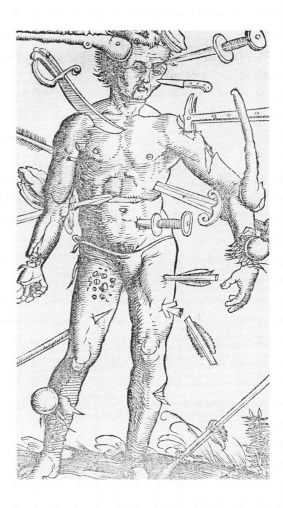

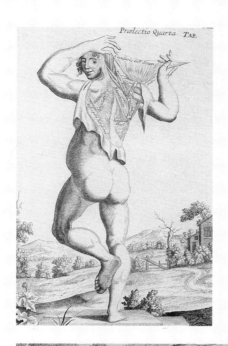

Anatomical plate from *Myographia Nova* by John Browne, 1697

John Browne (1642-1702) began his career as a surgeon in the navy and moved to London in the mid-1670s from Norwich. He became Surgeon-in-Ordinary to The King and surgeon to St Thomas's Hospital. The *Myographia Nova* was Browne's most popular work, although it was almost totally plagiarised from other authors. It contains 37 full-page engravings. The plagiarisms were revealed several years after their publication by James Young, who described Browne's work as 'twice sodden Cabbage, nothing new, nothing his own'. This illustration shows the superficial muscles of the back copied from an earlier Italian work and given a rural English background. The wry smile with which the jaunty figure holds open his own skin makes this illustration particularly appealing.

From *Tabulae Sceleti et Musculorum* by Bernard Seigfried Albinus, 1777

The *Tabulae* of Albinus (1697-1770) has been described as 'one of the most artistically perfect of all the anatomical atlases'. Albinus and his artist, Jan Wandelaar, used some ingenious methods to prepare the illustrations, including the establishment of an optically ideal point of view. In addition Wandelaar placed his skeletons and musclemen against lush ornamental backgrounds to give them an air of vitality. The most famous plate in the atlas shows a skeletal figure standing in front of an enormous grazing rhinoceros, which Wandelaar had sketched at the Amsterdam zoo from the first living specimen in Europe. Because the rhinoceros had never before been portrayed in European art from a living creature, Albinus and Wandelaar adopted it as a symbol of their atlas.

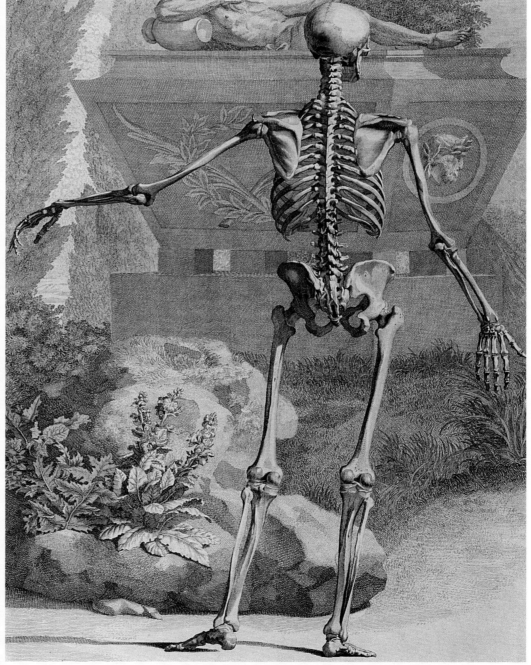

From *Drawings of Surgical Cases*
by Sir Astley Paston Cooper, 1814

This painting of a child with a hare-lip is taken from a
unique collection of drawings made by Cooper (1768-
1841). By all accounts a charming and handsome man,
Cooper became the King's personal surgeon and has
been described as one of the fathers of modern vascular
surgery. He attended John Hunter's lectures and was
greatly influenced by Hunter's methodical approach.
In spite of rarely getting home before midnight after
his last rounds, he used to wake his laboratory assistant
before sunrise so that he could undertake sufficient
dissections before breakfast. He used to say that a day
spent without dissection was a day lost!

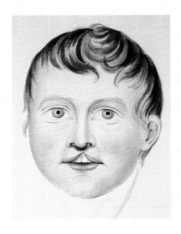

A Treatise on the Physiology and Diseases
of the Eye **by John Harrison Curtis, 1833**

Although this figure appeared in an ophthalmic text,
Curtis (1778-1860) started out working on the ear,
setting up the Dispensary for Diseases of the Ear in
1816. He had no formal medical qualifications. A man
of forceful personality, he married a lady of means and
social standing and managed to gain royal patronage.
In spite of his great success, Curtis' books are full of
inconsistencies; after attending a paper given by Curtis
in 1837 at the Medical Society of London, Joseph
Toynbee vowed 'to rescue aural surgery from the hands
of quacks'.

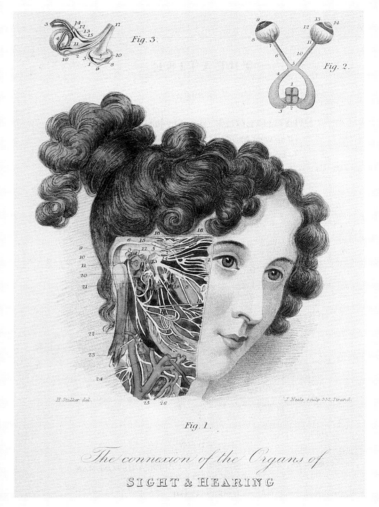

From *Traité Complete de L'anatomie*
de L'homme **by Jean-Baptiste Marc Bourgery,**
1831-54

Bourgery's atlas is noteworthy for the stunning hand-
coloured plates drawn by the artist Nicolas-Henri Jacob
(1782-1871) and transferred by a team of skilled
lithographers. Jacob had been a pupil of Jacques-Louis
David, the neo-classical artist of the French revolution,
and something of David's style can be seen in this plate,
which is entitled 'Elaborate compressors to occlude facial
and carotid arteries'. It is considered a superb drawing,
although it contains 'little evidence of practical value'.

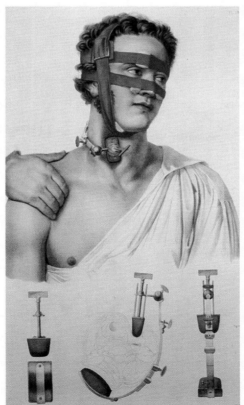

From *Osteographia or the Anatomy of the Bones* **by William Cheselden, 1733**

This outstanding book was considered in its time to be 'the most magnificent work of its kind'. In it Cheselden fully and accurately describes all the bones of the human body and many animal ones. Some of these bones are placed beautifully in context, for example, a confrontation between the skeleton of a cat and that of a mouse or the skeleton of a crocodile posed in front of the Pyramids. Cheselden was the first to use a camera obscura to give precision to his work. Cheselden was pre-eminent not only in orthopaedics but also in ophthalmology. Among his famous patients was Alexander Pope, who wrote:

> Weak tho' I am of limb and short of sight,
> Far from a lynx, and not a giant quite,
> I'll do what Mead and Cheseldon advise,
> To keep these limbs and to preserve these eyes.

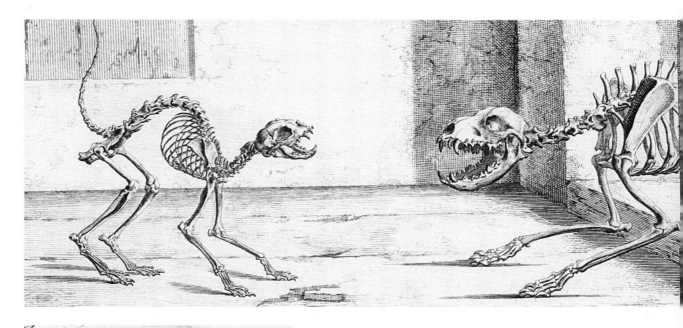

Illumination from the first page of *Opus Pandectarum Medicinae...* **by Matthaeus Silvaticus, 1474**

The book is a superb example of an incunabula (books printed before 1500).

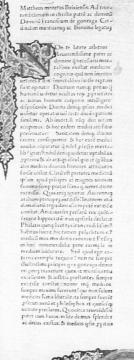

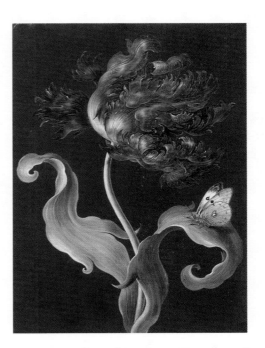

Painting of a tulip from the Hunter–Baillie Collection

It was long assumed to have been the work of a member of the famous Dietsch family of artists, but recent research casts doubt on this attribution.

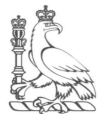

CHAPTER 17

The Museums and Special Collections: The College Heritage

The Museums

The 1941 photograph of Sir Arthur Keith (Fig 17.1 and see also Fig 4.25) and his assistant digging through the rubble of the College museum is very evocative. The Conservator is watched by the remains of Alfred Gilbert's bronze sculpture of Sir Richard Owen (see also Fig 3.23), the man who coined the word 'dinosaur' in 1841 and who created in the College a precursor to a national natural history museum. The reduction of the vast museum galleries to a pile of bricks and twisted metal was a disaster. For nearly 150 years the story of the Museum had been inseparable from that of the College: Hunter's collection had been acquired at the time when the Company was transforming itself into a College of Surgeons and surgery in London was emerging as a respectable profession.

After Owen, the reputation of the Museum attracted other giants in the museum profession (and in science), among them Sir William Flower, John Quekett, Professor Charles Stewart and Keith himself. Nevertheless, by 1939 many felt that the Museum was holding back the development of the College, that it was a museum with a College attached. At the outbreak of the Second World War, Council considered the transfer of non-medical material to the British Museum (Natural History). After the war, there was an opportunity to examine the role of the surviving material from the Hunterian Collection, the Odontological Collection and the other specimen collections. Comparative anatomy and pathology were no longer central to surgical and dental training but remained relevant to the work of the research departments within the College, including the Buckston Browne Farm at Downe. Basic surgical training still required dissected specimens of human anatomy and pathology. Important prehistoric and fossil material, including most of the surviving specimens given to the Museum by Charles Darwin, were transferred to the British

Museum (Natural History). Hunter's own collection, although reduced to 3,500 original specimens, endured as an icon for the College and the surgical profession. It was decided, therefore, to divide the museum collections according to purpose into four galleries in different locations within the rebuilt College.

The near simultaneous rebuilding of the Hunterian Museum with the College was thanks to the energy of the Board of Trustees of the Hunterian Collection and a generous grant from the Wolfson Foundation. In a letter pledging support, the Wolfson Foundation in 1961 expressed the belief that 'The Hunterian Museum is the key centre of The Royal College of Surgeons and [is] probably the finest of its kind in the world.'

17.1 Sir Arthur Keith in the ruins of the Museum

During the Second World War, books, paintings and other College treasures were removed to the country for safety, while the specimens were packed in the basement and sub-basement of the College. When the Museum suffered a direct hit, fire penetrated into the basements and devastated the collection. Keith was Conservator of the Collection, as had been Sir Richard Owen. Keith attracted students from all over the world and made the Museum a centre for research in anatomy and anthropology. The bronze bust of Owen was repaired and is on display in the Hunterian Museum.

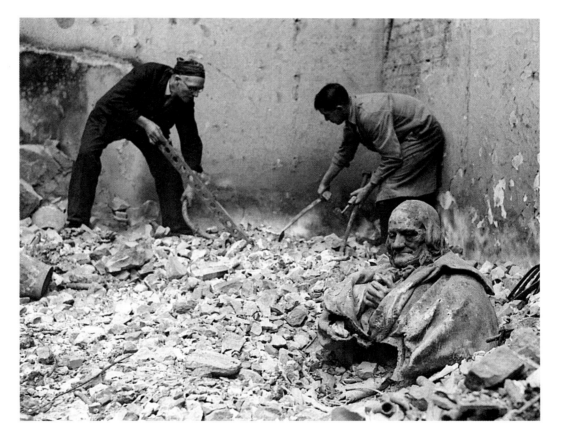

Support from the Wellcome Trust helped establish museums of anatomy and pathology, which provided valuable resources for the research work and teaching of their respective departments. From the 1950s through to the 1980s, all the museums served the many researchers and trainees who were based at, or visited, the College. In turn, research work shed new light on many of the historic specimens.

During the 1980s, a Museums Conservation Unit was established to care for the specimen collections in the College (Fig 17.2). Until that time, specimens had been maintained by technicians and by a prosector attached to the departments of anatomy and pathology. The Conservation Unit operating in this unique environment has since developed into a centre of museum expertise, which today is recognised all over the world.

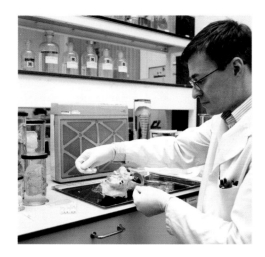

17.2 Martyn Cooke, Head of the Museums Conservation Unit

In 1993 the College joined with the Trustees of the Hunterian Collection to celebrate the bicentenary of the death of John Hunter and to reflect on Hunter's contributions to the College and to the profession of surgery. After a memorial service in St Margaret's Church, Westminster, Sir Miles Irving gave the biennial Hunterian Oration in which he described Hunter's continuing influence:

> We can regard Hunter's legacy of surgical science and practice as a baton to be passed on as in a relay race through time....passed from Hunter through successive generations of surgeons by taking as an example the studies undertaken primarily by surgeons, and those working in close collaboration with them, on physiology, metabolism and clinical management of injury, and on the organisation and delivery of services for the injured.

By registering its museums with the Museums and Galleries Commission, the College ensured that they maintain basic standards of service and collection care and provide appropriate public access (Fig 17.3). The Hunterian and Odontological Museums are open to the public without charge on weekdays when the College is open. Public interest in the history of medicine has never been stronger, encouraged largely through the work of the Wellcome Institute for the History of Medicine as well as the work of social historians and the media in this area. As the most famous private 18th century museum of comparative anatomy with supporting artefacts, paintings and archives, the Hunterian Museum is an important part of the story of medicine. Historic material given later to the Museum also indicates that its value is wider than the history of the surgical and dental profession: it appeals to biologists, veterinary surgeons, artists, anthropologists and historians.

17.3 Members of the public visiting the Hunterian Museum during a College Open Evening in 1996

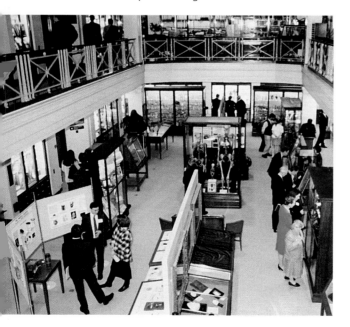

The Museum now provides the focus for many public activities – National Science Week, Heritage Open House weekends and College Open Days. Staff contribute to national and local initiatives to rescue pathology collections, raise the profile of medical collections and offer professional curatorial training. The Honorary Curator of Historic Surgical Instruments is called upon by museums, auction houses, collectors and the media to identify instruments and provide expert advice.

The Museums of Anatomy and Pathology are available to medical, dental and related students and all healthcare professionals. There are plans to incorporate digitised images of the specimens in the production of computer-aided learning programmes: specimens will become a reference library underpinning College courses and self-directed study. Surgeons can be seen brushing up on their knowledge on a particular area of anatomy, and overseas doctors are frequent users of the Pathology Museum. Although the direct use of specimens may decline in the future, the facility to view and study real anatomical and pathological specimens will remain a valuable resource for basic and continuing medical education.

The Board of Trustees of the Hunterian Collection

The establishment of the Board of Trustees to supervise the care and maintenance of the Hunterian Collection predates the College by a few months. Thirty Trustees were appointed by the government of William Pitt, 16 by virtue of their office. The other 14 seats were appointed in 1799 but afterwards were filled by election. The original Board of Trustees comprised:

Trustees by Office: The Lord Chancellor; The First Lord of the Treasury; The Chancellor of the Exchequer; The First Lord of the Admiralty; The Speaker of the House of Commons; The Secretary at War; President of the Royal Society; President of the Royal College of Physicians; The four Censors of the Royal College of Physicians; The Regius Professor of Medicine in the University of Oxford; The Reader in Anatomy in the University of Oxford;

Sir Reginald Murley, Chairman of the Trustees 1988–96 (see also Fig 6.22), guiding Her Majesty The Queen around the Hunterian Museum

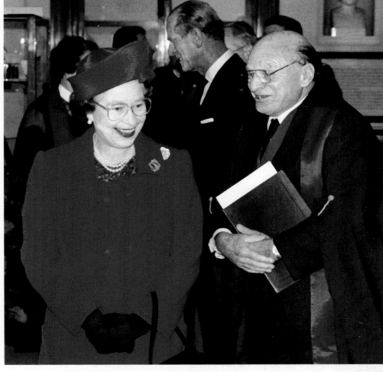

The Regius Professor of Physic in the University of Cambridge; The Professor of Anatomy in the University of Cambridge.

Trustees by Appointment: Lord Auckland; Earl of Euston; George Rose; Charles Small Pybus; Matthew Baillie; Lord St Helen; Lord Arden; Sir Charles Blagden; Isaac Hawkins Browne; Sir Archibald Macdonald; The Bishop of Llandaff; Edward Whitaker Gray; Charles Long; Sir George Shuckleburgh Evelyn.

Over the last 200 years its composition has changed very little. In 1856 the President of The Royal College of Surgeons was added as a Trustee by Office. In 1921 the Oxford University's Reader in Anatomy was replaced by Dr Lee's Professor of Anatomy. In 1964 the offices of First Lord of the Admiralty and the Secretary at War were abolished and they were not replaced on the Board. Today the membership of the elected Trustees reflects close links with the College, surgery and museums.

It is fascinating to look back in the archives and see the business of the Trustees. Making the collection accessible to visitors through tours and the production of catalogues has been a continuing priorty, as has the provision of adequate accommodation. Of less interest now is the acquisition of new material (human and animal); today this has been replaced by concern to conserve and preserve the unique material. As a new redisplay of the collection is planned, an active partnership between the Board of Trustees and the College will ensure that the Hunterian Collection survives for another century.

The Hunterian Museum

Of John Hunter's original collection, 3,500 specimens have survived (Figs 17.4–17.7). The essential fragility of much of the material – pieces of bone and tissue suspended by thin thread and housed in glass vessels full of highly flammable liquid – makes its survival all the more miraculous. The thrill of seeing the two-tailed lizard collected by Hunter when a young army surgeon in Portugal in 1762 or the alizarin-stained seven-week-old foetus is heightened by awareness of its vulnerability and of Hunter's skilful methods of preparation.

The present Hunterian Museum was planned by Frederic Wood Jones, Professor of Anatomy and Conservator of the Museum (see also Fig 5.8), and the Curator, Jessie Dobson, to follow the order outlined in John Hunter's own catalogue and as published in Dobson's catalogue of 1972–74. All original Hunterian specimens of the physiological and reproductive series were placed on the ground floor, together with some replacements to supplement certain sections where little original material had survived. The sections demonstrate Hunter's theories about the form and function of plants and animals: their locomotion, digestion, circulation and reproduction. The range of species included and the quality of the preparations still instruct and fascinate. A Surinam toad is shown at the very moment the young toads can be seen emerging and crawling over her back. In another, the human spinal cord ending is unravelled to show the strands as a horse's tail.

Hunter's surviving pathology specimens are located at the end of the lower gallery. The pathology section illustrates some of the common conditions of 18th century Londoners, from syphilis to poorly healed fractures. Here can be found some of the most celebrated of Hunter's specimens, such as the earliest surviving recorded specimen of metastasis, in this case of the lung, the popliteal aneurysm and the large parotid tumour successfully excised by Hunter and recorded in his casebook. The upper gallery continues the same arrangement but uses surviving specimens from the post-Hunter collections, including specimens prepared by Richard Owen and William Flower.

In between these central themes, additional items and specimens of interest are exhibited. These, like Hunter's dental material and commissioned animal paintings, are essential ingredients of the Hunter story or, like John Evelyn's *Anatomical Tables* and the wax anatomical models by Joseph Towne, part of the history of the Museum and the College.

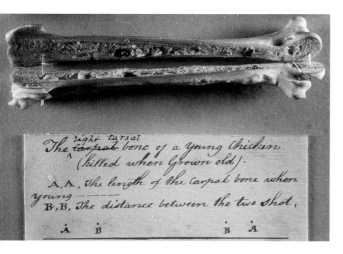

17.4 Bone growth

Hunter demonstrated growth sites in bone by inserting two pieces of lead shot into a young chicken's leg and by measuring the distance between the lead shots and overall length of bone at the start of the experiment and after a period of growth.

17.5 The didine moa – an extinct bird from New Zealand

When, in 1839, Richard Owen was shown a shaft of bone from New Zealand that resembled an ox's marrow bone, he deduced that it was part of the femur of a huge, flightless, ostrich-like bird unknown to science and drew a predictive sketch of the whole bone. Later, in 1843, when sufficient bones had been collected to reassemble a complete skeleton, Owen's predictions of the size and form of the bird were shown to be correct. The museum specimen of a didine moa *(Anomalopteryx didiformis)*, presented by Dr Julius von Haast in 1873, was articulated using William Flower's modified technique, so that the skeleton could be taken apart easily without damage. Another species *(A. maximus)* grew to over ten feet tall.

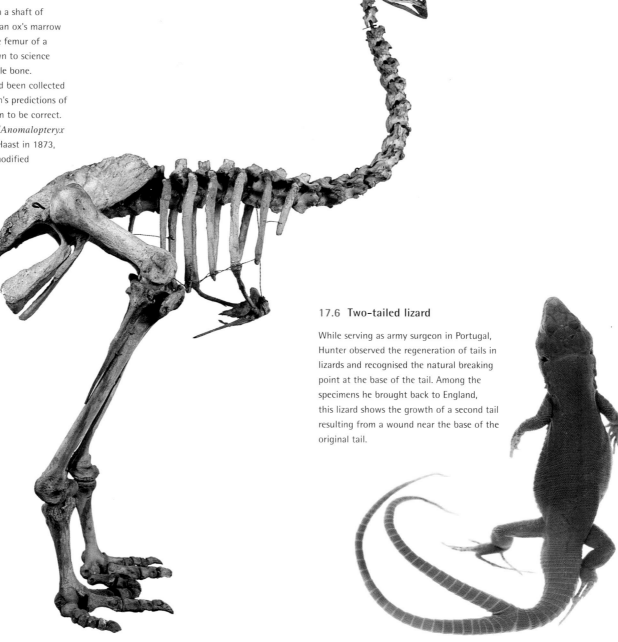

17.6 Two-tailed lizard

While serving as army surgeon in Portugal, Hunter observed the regeneration of tails in lizards and recognised the natural breaking point at the base of the tail. Among the specimens he brought back to England, this lizard shows the growth of a second tail resulting from a wound near the base of the original tail.

17.7 Treatment of popliteal aneurysm

Hunter's greatest contribution to operative surgery was his management of popliteal aneurysm, a condition common in coachmen. This was a potentially fatal disease of the artery behind the knee, for which the usual treatment was amputation of the leg above the knee. Hunter, having already demonstrated the development of a collateral circulation, tied the femoral artery in the thigh to relieve pressure on the weakened wall and partially blocked vessel in the expectation that the collateral circulation would restore an adequate blood supply to the lower limb. Although the first three operations were successful, the patients died of some unrelated disease within a few years. His fourth patient, a coachman, survived with a healthy leg for 50 years and outlived Hunter.

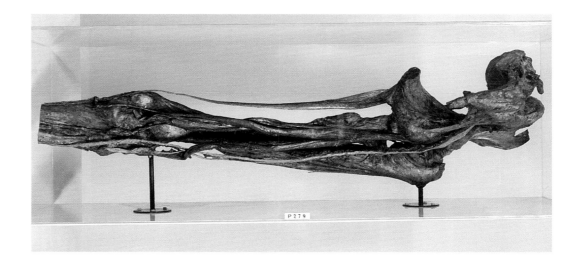

Odontological Museum

The Odontological Collection is to dentistry what the Hunterian Collection is to surgery. The fact that all 10,000 specimens survived the war-time devastation underlines its value as a complete historic collection (Fig 17.8).

17.8 Twisted elephant trunk

This spiral tusk from an African elephant *(Loxodonta africana)* was donated to the Royal Society by Thomas Crispe of the Royal African Society before 1681 and exhibited in their museum at Gresham College. The College eventually purchased it from the British Museum in 1809. This specimen is part of a special highlights display in the Odontological Museum.

The museum began life as the Museum of the Odontological Society for the Advancement of Science in Dental Surgery. This society was formed in 1856 primarily to campaign for the formal examination of dental surgeons by the College. Their campaign succeeded; in 1860 the first dental examinations were held in the College. The members of this learned society met to discuss examples and cases using specimens or casts. By 1859, the collection of specimens used for these discussions was large enough to be called a museum. In 1863 the rival College of Dentists and its museum were absorbed into the Society, which itself was absorbed into the Royal Society of Medicine in 1907. The collections were transferred to the care of the College in 1909, first on loan and later, in 1943, as a gift.

At its core is the collection of Sir John Tomes. Tomes (see also Fig 13.1) carried out pioneering research into the structure of teeth following on from Hunter's work. He was co-founder and first Secretary of the Odontological Society, and became the first President of the British Dental Association in 1880. The Tomes' collection of human skulls and jaws of known sex and age with some clinical history provided a benchmark for dental and anthropological studies. Specimens include rare examples of necrosis of the jaw, an industrial disease caused by exposure to yellow phosphorous during the manufacture of matches (Fig 17.9). The sheer technical skill

17.9 'Phossy' jaw

Damage to the jaw due to phosphorus necrosis of the bone was a high industrial risk to match makers in the 19th century. Although the cause was recognised in 1844, it was not until 1910 that legislation prohibiting the use of 'white phosphorus' in British match factories was enacted. The specimen was donated by Sir John Tomes.

involved with preparing the specimens could not be reproduced today, and dentists still marvel at some of these specimens.

As with the Hunterian Museum, there are some fascinating items in addition to Tomes' collection, such as WAN Cattlin's specimens displaying the maxillary antrum. Cattlin was one of the first to take the dental examination at the College. The specimens were illustrated in his paper on the maxillary antrum presented to the Odontological Society in 1858. Also unique is the collection of specimens of dental disease and abnormalities in animals, which brings together examples from species (such as elephants, lions, boars and a large number of primates) now on the endangered list. One of the more recent additions is a collection of 230 Anglo-Saxon skulls excavated at Breedon-on-the-Hill and Polhill (Fig 17.10). They show examples of disease such as osteomyelitis and examples of trauma.

17.10 Skull c. 600 taken from an Anglo Saxon burial ground at Breedon-on-the-Hill, Leicestershire

Approximately 190 individuals were identified from the excavated material, and their remains were used by Professor AEW Miles to construct a system for assessing the relative ages at death of individuals according to the degree of tooth wear.

In general, teeth are not the most attractive items for display, although certain animal skulls and some human specimens are of great visual interest. For the lay visitor, the amount of graphic interpretation necessary to point out the context or value of the specimens on display would outweigh the space available. Today the collection is essentially a reference tool for dentists, veterinarians and anthropologists. Still, in choosing what to show, the challenge is to balance scientific value with historic significance.

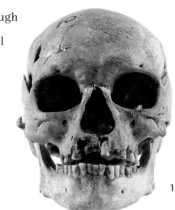

17.10

Museums of Anatomy and Pathology

The Anatomy Museum contains some 600 examples of human anatomy arranged according to regions of the body. Specimens include a complete body in transverse sections. The specimens are supported by X-rays, histological slides and the unique Tompsett resin casts of blood vessels, tracheo-bronchial trees, biliary and urinary tracts and ventricles of the brain (Fig 17.11). Some 20 years on these casts are now historical, and with the resin decaying they will provide an interesting task for the Museums Conservation Unit.

In spite of the amount of anatomical teaching material available on the Internet these specimens continue to be useful, particularly in self-study. Specimens are brought out when courses are held so that trainees can check the anatomy while working on particular procedures (Fig 17.12).

The Pathology Museum contains about 2,500 specimens collected from the 19th century to the present day. The material is arranged systematically, with more common conditions distinguished from specimens showing extreme or rare manifestations. Many of the diseases listed as extinct are making an unwelcome return, and the more historical of the pathological specimens may be the only way doctors can examine these conditions.

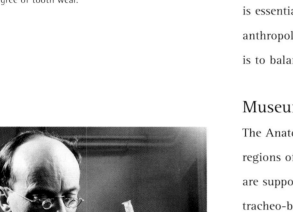

17.11 David Tompsett and his corrosion casts

David Tompsett, a skilled prosector who worked in the anatomy department from 1944 to 1977, revived the 18th century technique of wax corrosion casting by using modern resins to produce excellent three-dimensional demonstrations of the arteries, veins or other vessels and cavities of the body in both animals and humans.

17.12 Dr Vishy Mahadevan, Barber Professor of Surgery, using specimens to assist teaching

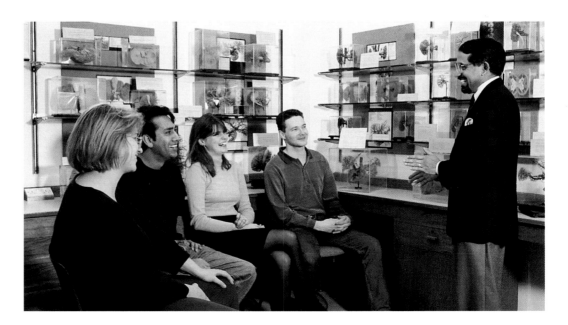

Historical Surgical Instruments

This important collection, started in 1804, was displayed in its own exhibition gallery in the pre-war museum. Sadly, irreplaceable instruments and equipment were destroyed in 1941, including almost all of Hunter's own instruments and a unique Roman bronze artificial leg. Since then, many donors have added to the collection, which now totals over 7,000 items varying from ethnological material and standard amputation and trephine sets, to the personal innovations and instruments of surgeons including Cheselden, Pott, Brodie, Spencer Wells, Macewen, Moynihan and Gillies (Figs 17.13 and 17.14).

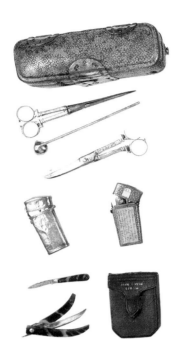

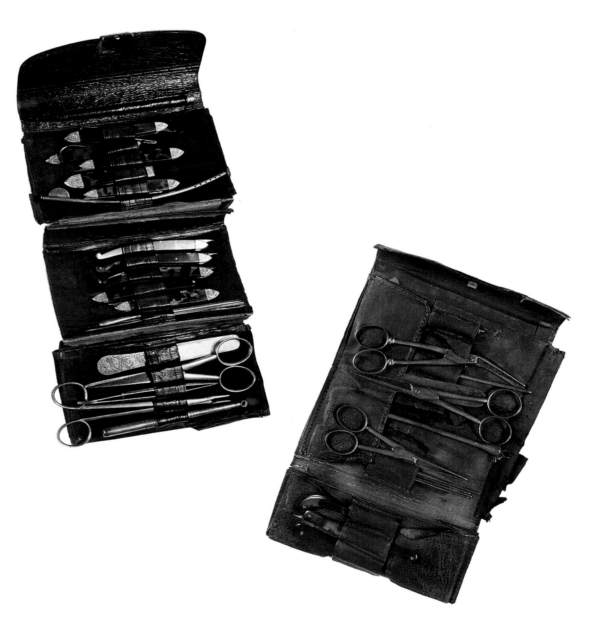

17.13 Pocket cases

From the 17th century, surgeons carried lancet cases in their waistcoats and minor instrument kits in their jacket pockets. This would explain how a surgeon incarcerated in the Black Hole of Calcutta, Mungo Park, was able to extricate himself from hostile hands: though he had lost everything else, he had lancets in his hidden instrument case. Thomas Dimsdale struck riches with his lancets in Russia, receiving £12,000, pensions and a baronetcy for treating the Empress of Russia.

above, top to bottom

Pocket case, all silver items except blades of scissors and forceps, 1672

Lancet case from the Black Hole of Calcutta, 1753

Dimsdale's lancet case employed to inoculate the Empress of Russia and her son, 1768

Hunter's minor instrument case c. 1790

middle

Park's well-worn case used in West Africa, 1795

right

Thomas Colledge's instrument case, tortoise shell and silver gilt, used in China c. 1859.

17.14 Instrument innovations

Many instruments have been devised or modernised by surgeons associated with the College; this selection notes the date of introduction.

left to right

Cheselden's eye speculum based on the spring forceps, c. 1730

Cooper's aneurysm needle used for over a century, c. 1795

Liston's linear bone-cutting forceps with curved blades still in use today, c. 1820

Durham's tracheal tube and lobster claw pilot, c. 1870

Wells' second arterial forceps, of which he said that elimination of the aperture between handles prevented entanglement with omentum, 1878

Mackenzie's tonsil guillotine with handle removed but swivelled for right and left use, before 1889

Moynihan's gastrectomy clamp with fenestrated jaws, c. 1900.

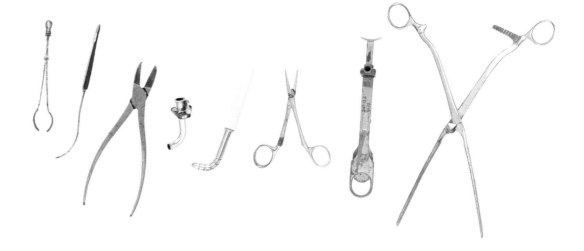

The outstanding donation remains Joseph Lister's research equipment, workbooks and water-colour drawings, as well as his surgical instruments, many of which he designed (Fig 17.15). Overall, the collection is rich in late 18th, 19th and early 20th century artefacts reflecting the instrument innovations associated with thermal sterilisation techniques and the introduction of stainless steel; it is, however, deficient in material from the second half of the 20th century.

17.15 Lister's collection

An extensive range of artefacts associated with Joseph Lister is on view in and around the commemorative Lister cabinet, constructed in 1924, now on display in the Hunterian Museum.

left to right

Lister's microscope made by his cousins, the Becks, c. 1865

Wiring for patellar fracture; thanks to safe antisepsis he pioneered the open reduction of fractures

Catgut preparation in phenol; Lister researched over 40 years to make catgut the first safe absorbable ligature material

Lister's dressing forceps

Carbolic acid steam spray, part of an antiseptic regime introduced 1870 and abandoned 1887.

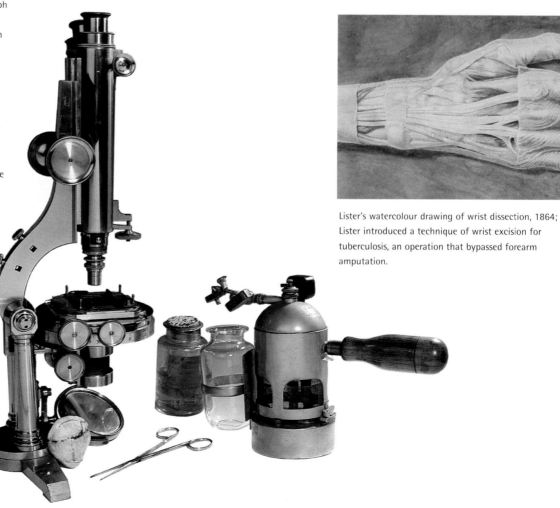

Lister's watercolour drawing of wrist dissection, 1864; Lister introduced a technique of wrist excision for tuberculosis, an operation that bypassed forearm amputation.

17.16 Bureau cabinet and painting

The walnut cabinet (c. 1720), now in the President's Lodge, formerly belonged to Joshua Ward, a well-known figure in early Georgian London. He was a 'quack' doctor and sold cure-all pills known as 'Ward's drops', a compound of antimony. He was caricatured by William Hogarth, but the College owns a painting by Thomas Bardwell that depicts Ward as a great benefactor of the sick poor. It shows an allegorical scene of Britannia presenting a group of patients to Ward who stands large and benign outside a classical building. Above Ward's head Time draws back a curtain as if to say that his place in history is assured. The cabinet was bequeathed to the College by Mrs Ada Lance in 1955 and the painting was bequeathed in 1945 by a descendent of Ward, Mrs C P E de H Larpent.

Furniture and Clocks

The collection of historical furniture and clocks (Figs 17.16–17.19) is derived primarily from two sources – donations (gifts and bequests) and furniture inherited from the Company or brought in by the College to furnish and decorate rooms. The collection is not large, but a number of items are of great historic interest. Sir John Bland-Sutton's exotic antiquarian taste can be seen in the items of furniture bequested to the College by his widow. These include chairs decorated with winged Assyrian gods, and a fireplace in the Egyptian style from his own house in Brook Street. At one time the whole of Committee Room 3 on the ground floor of the College, called the Bland-Sutton Room, was furnished with items from his collection. When the houses at 44 and 45 Lincoln's Inn Fields were demolished to make way for the Imperial Cancer Research Fund Headquarters in the early 1960s, some fine examples of carved Georgian woodwork were saved and brought into the College.

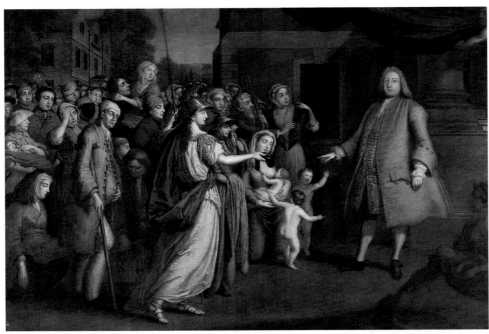

17.16b

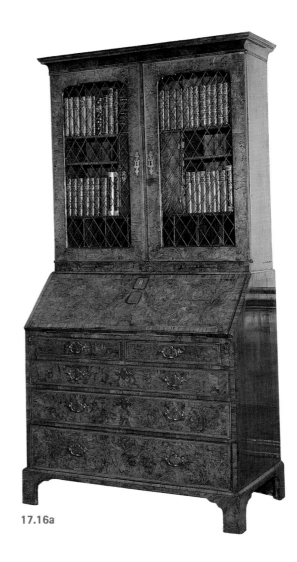

17.16a

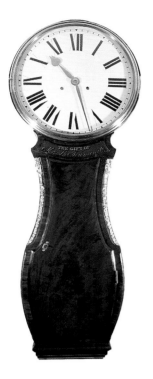

17.17 Company of Surgeons' wall clock

This mahogany clock was given to the Company of Surgeons in 1765 by John Townsend, Master of the Company in 1762. His gift is recorded in the minutes of the Court of Assistants.

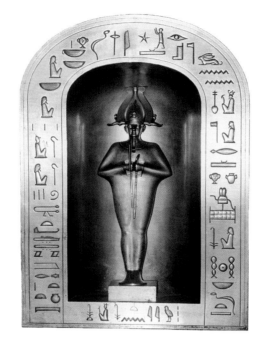

17.18 Architectural decoration in the Egyptian style

This brass item is part of the Bland-Sutton bequest, which also includes a fireplace, chairs, bureaux and light fittings.

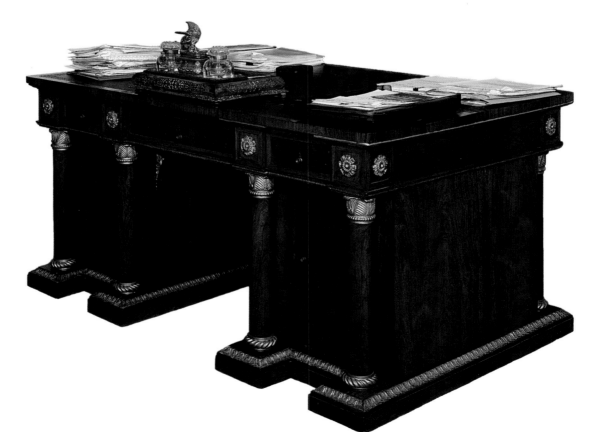

17.19 Pedestal desk c. 1825

One of the most important items in the furniture collection is this desk currently used by the President. Dating from the Regency period, it is a rare English rosewood and brass inlaid pedestal library desk, made in the manner of Louis Légaigneur.

Silver

The College's silver collection is small but varied. With its contents reflecting the individual taste of various donors, it will be fascinating to see how it develops in the future (Figs 17.20–17.22).

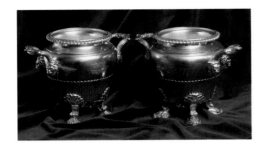

17.20 Wine coolers

Paul Storr, probably one of the most famous of London silversmiths, made this pair of silver wine coolers in 1815. They are typical of his work. Presented by the Faculty of Ophthalmologists in 1950.

17.21 Cheselden Cup

Silver gilt cup and cover similar in shape to the Ranby Cup but much simpler. It is engraved with the arms of the Cheseldens of Uppingham, Rutland and was made by John Bignell, London, 1725.

17.22 Bland-Sutton condiment set

Sir John and Lady Bland-Sutton gave many pieces of silver but this condiment set is the most spectacular. Made by David J Welby of London in 1910, the set consists of 70 pieces, all in Assyrian style:

left to right

Lion (for mustard)
Warrior (to hold flowers)
Two-headed bull (for salt)
Priest (for pepper)
Lotus leaf container (for nuts)
Doorway (menu holders)
Arrow-shaped spoon

The Worshipful Company of Barbers possesses well-known pieces of silver from early surgical history, and in 1950 presented to the College a replica of Henry VIII's Grace Cup made by Elkington & Co in 1895 (see also Fig 1.8). A replica of Charles II's Boscobel Cup by Wakely & Wheeler was given to the College by Lord Brock on relinquishing the office of President in 1960. Presidents have added a number of interesting items of contemporary silver. A few pieces were inherited from the Company of Surgeons, including the Company mace and the Ranby Cup (see also Fig 2.1). Some items have been given because of their association with a famous surgeon, for example Hunter's Tankard (see also Fig 2.7a) and the Cheselden Cup (Fig 17.21).

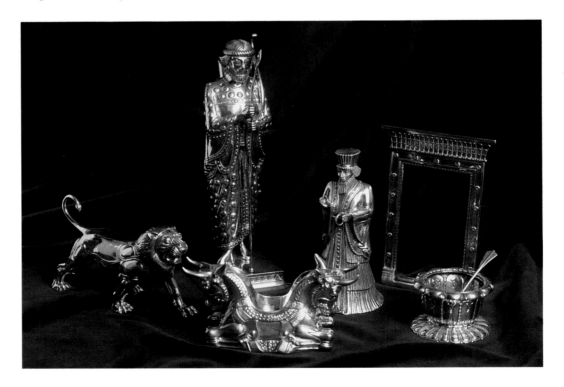

17.21

The largest single donation of silver was a 70-piece condiment set made for the dining table of Sir John and Lady Bland-Sutton in their house in Brook Street (Fig 17.22). The set, left to the College on Lady Bland-Sutton's death in 1943, makes regular appearances at College functions.

Ceramics

Drug jars are some of the most attractive items of medical history (Figs 17.23–17.26). They were functional and commonplace, yet colourful and imaginatively decorated. The regional forms and decorative traditions make them extremely collectible, and the College has a small but representative number. A large part of the collection was bequeathed by Sir St Clair Thomson in 1943. A few additional jars and other pieces, such as barber's bowls and pill slabs, were added later.

The collection comprises coloured Italian and Spanish Majolica dating from the 16th–18th centuries, and blue and white Delftware from Northern Europe dating from the 17th–19th centuries. The group of Delftware from London is especially interesting; they range from tiny pots for ointment and lozenges to elegant jars with spouts for syrups, distillations and oils. The large cylindrical jars often stored bulky dried plant material. The tops were usually sealed with parchment caps.

17.23 Italian Majolica

left to right

Faenza jar c. 1560, labelled for conserve of senna

Jar with cover from Castelli, Abruzzo, 2nd half of 17th century, decorated with the coat-of-arms of the Holy Roman Empire. Labelled for vinegar and honey of squills.

17.24 Delftware from England – London

left to right

Dry drug jar, c.1652, for the Universal Purge

Wet drug jar, 1669, for syrup of roses with senna

Oviform jar, 1672, for lozenges of aloes, ambergris and musk.

17.25 Delftware from England – London

left to right

Cylindrical jar, c. 1700 for confection of roses

Oviform jar, early 18th century, for rhubarb pills

Globular jar, mid-18th century, for syrup of lemon juice.

17.26 Chinese ceramic bowl of the *famille rose* design c. 1760s and decorated with the arms of the Company of Surgeons

17.23

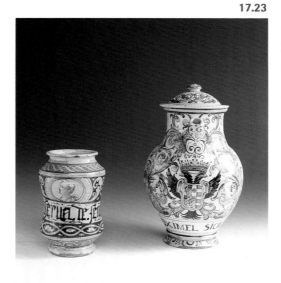

17.24

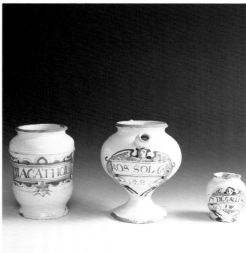

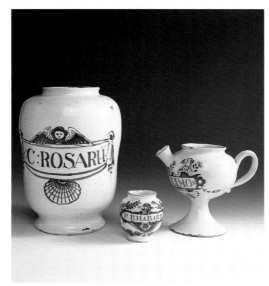

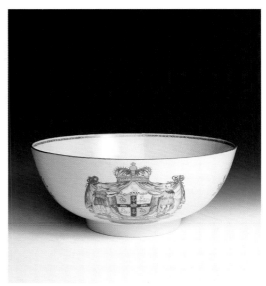

17.25

17.26

Fine Art

The richness of the College's art collection is surprising (Figs 17.27–17.33). Paintings and sculpture are scattered around the building as decoration, with the result that they are not seen as a significant whole. Drawings and prints are kept out of the light for conservation reasons, and the lack of an exhibition space together with increasing commercial use of the rooms prevents them from being regularly displayed.

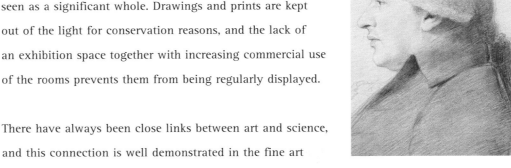

17.27

There have always been close links between art and science, and this connection is well demonstrated in the fine art collection. There are portraits of surgeons by some of the leading portrait artists of their day: Hans Holbein, William Hogarth, George Dance, Joseph Nollekens, George Richmond, Sir Thomas Lawrence, Sir Francis Chantrey and Sir Jacob Epstein. Many artists of the 18th and 19th centuries attended anatomical lectures and made the acquaintance of surgeons and anatomists, as in recent times Dame Barbara Hepworth attended the operations of Norman Capener (see also Fig 15.7). Surgeons often commissioned artists to draw specimens or to paint people and animals with unusual conditions. Some surgeons learnt to draw in order to record material for scientific or artistic reasons. The collection also includes depictions of the history of the College and the evolution of its building in Lincoln's Inn Fields.

Portraits – Paintings, Drawings and Sculpture

Portraits of distinguished past members of the College dominate the art collection. Many of the well-known portraits featured elsewhere in this book illustrate the achievements of the sitter, as in the portrait by William Hogarth (1697–1764) of his friend Sir Caesar Hawkins (see also Fig 2.9); others represent a significant event in the evolution of the College, such as the overpainted cartoon (see also Fig 1.9) by Hans Holbein (1460–1524).

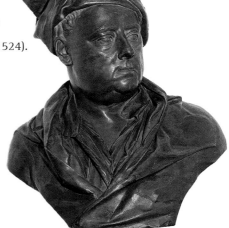

17.27

In 1898, the College purchased a series of drawings by George Dance (1740–1825) depicting a number of leading surgeons of the 1790s. The drawings, in pencil tinted with crayon, have been kept out of sunlight and appear fresh and full of character. Dance made over 200 portrait drawings in this profile style; he made portraits of the leading surgeons of the day as well as musicians, actors, lawyers, politicians among other sections of Georgian London's middle-class and gentry. The drawing of Sir James Earle, Serjeant-Surgeon to King George III and Master of the College in 1807, exemplifies the qualities of the group.

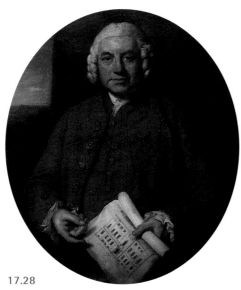

17.28

Nathanial Dance, George Dance's brother, painted a dramatic portrait of William Bromfeild, who was Master of the Company of Surgeons in 1769. Bromfeild is seen pointing to a plan of the London Lock Hospital for venereal diseases, which he founded in 1743. The painting was acquired in 1953 from the Paddington Group Hospital Management Committee.

17.29

Louis Francois Roubiliac (1695–1762) was one of the leading monument sculptors working in London in the mid-18th century. His terracotta bust of William Cheselden, Master of the Company in 1746, is one of the most important works of art in the collection and was presented to the College by William Lucas, a Master of the Company of Surgeons, in 1804.

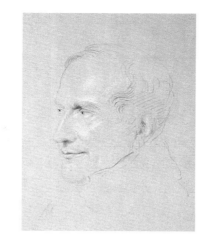

17.30

Sir William Lawrence was President of the College in 1846 and 1855. The College possesses portraits of him in oils and sculpture, but this crayon drawing by John Linnell (1792–1882), purchased in 1954, reveals a directness not possible in formal representations.

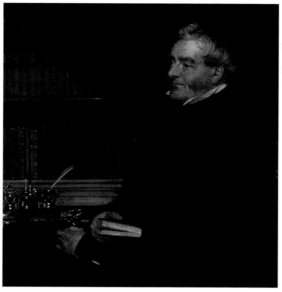

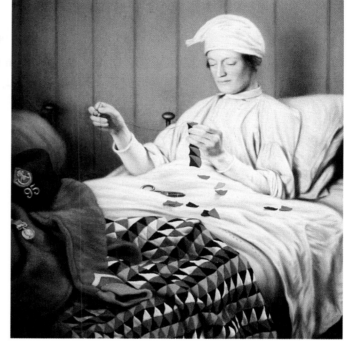

17.31

Charles Robert Leslie's small portrait of Benjamin Travers, President of the College in 1847 and 1875, bequeathed by Miss Travers in 1902, represents the best in 19th century portraiture. It is dignified but shows a warmth and humanity not always present in the stiff, dark portraits by some of his contemporaries.

17.32

Portraits of patients are rare and tend to be representations of the condition, injury or pathology. The colourful portrait of Private Thomas Walker – painted by Thomas Wood in 1856 – is an exception to all the rules. Walker was wounded in the head at the Battle of Inkerman in 1854. He underwent a successful trephining operation and was seen by Queen Victoria when she visited the Fort Pitt Military Hospital in 1855. He is shown sitting up in bed and working on a patchwork quilt made from uniform pieces. This portrait is more famous among quilt-makers than it is among surgeons.

17.33

One of the most extraordinary examples of portrait sculpture is the memorial to Edward Macloghlin (1855–1904) and his wife Eliza (1863–1928) who commissioned it from Sir Alfred Gilbert. It was presented to the College in 1909 by Mrs Macloghlin, who also funded the Carrara marble floor in 1911 and established educational scholarships. It is considered one of Gilbert's best works, but it is an unusual item to have in the College in that it contains the subjects' ashes.

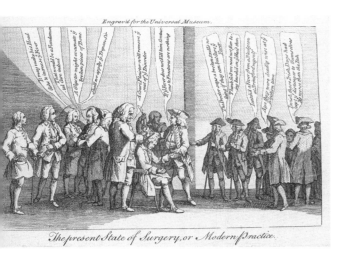

17.34 A typical 18th century caricature on surgeons

Caricatures and Genre Scenes

Caricatures of medical practitioners and patients have been popular for centuries and have been enthusiastically collected by the practitioners themselves (Fig 17.34). In England this reached new heights with the work of Thomas Rowlandson (1756–1827). The College is fortunate in owning four original watercolours, which were engraved and published as prints, namely: The Irish Giant, The Dissecting Room (see also Fig 2.5), John Heaviside Lecturing at Surgeons' Hall (see also Fig 2.8) and The Resurrectionists (see also Fig 3.14). They reflected the public's general anxiety about the activities of anatomists. The College print collection includes a number of coloured engravings and lithographs poking fun at the College or surgery and medical education in general.

There are very few representations of surgeons at work as there has been no active collecting in this area. Those that are in the collection are important in terms of artist and subject. Henry Tonks made several drawings of Harold Gillies at work (see also Fig 4.21) and Anna Zinkeisen's drawing on tracing paper shows Archibald McIndoe at work during the Second World War (see also Fig 5.10). Both artists were primarily in attendance to draw treatment and specimens.

Sir Roy Calne paints patients and self-portraits of himself operating (Fig 17.35). The College recently acquired three drawings by Julia Midgley made while she was artist in residence at the Royal Liverpool & Broadgreen Hospitals Trust (Fig 17.36).

17.35 Operation Scene

By Sir Roy Calne

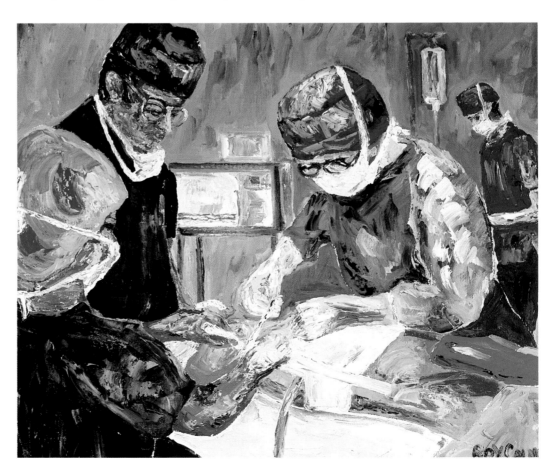

17.36 On Video

By Julia Midgley

Barbara Hepworth became acquainted with Norman Capener during the Second World War. In 1947 they met again, and Hepworth arranged to visit the Princess Elizabeth Orthopaedic Hospital at Exeter to see the surgeons at work. She made numerous ink sketches, which were exhibited in London. Capener presented one of her pictures to the College in 1969 (Fig 17.37). He records that:

> After the exhibition in 1948 I gave the artist two rather long panels of old pine wood. These she joined sideways and in the resulting picture [Concourse], which is pure oil painting, she appears to have summed up the whole experience. It was the last and largest production in this series of operating theatre pictures.

17.37 Concourse

By Barbara Hepworth

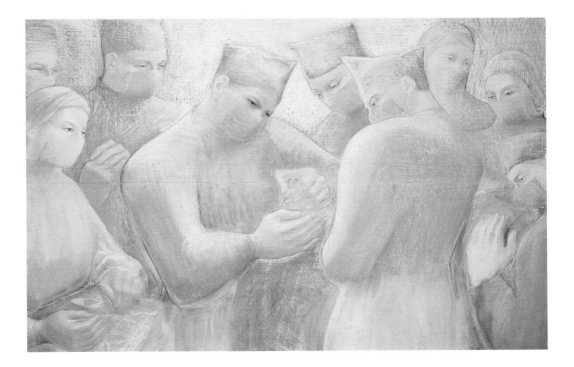

The Hunterian Art Collection

The College houses the paintings that were hanging in John Hunter's museum at the time of his death (Figs 17.38–17.42). Hunter had a large collection of paintings, drawings, watercolours and prints in a separate gallery in his house, but they were sold at Christies in 1794. The present Hunterian Art Collection includes three paintings by George Stubbs (1724–1806) and portraits by William Hodges (1744–1797) and the American artist Benjamin West (1738–1820). John Hunter employed artists to record his specimens and people of interest and to illustrate his books. Jan van Rymsdyk (active 1750–1784) was one whose work survives in the

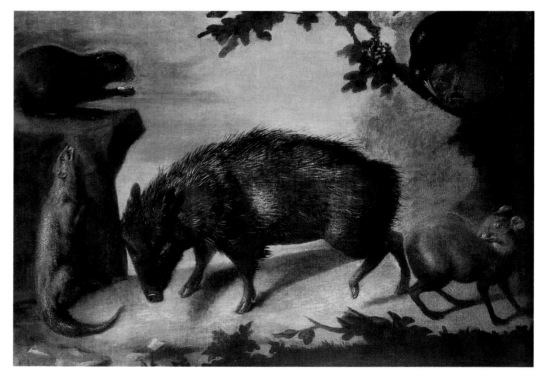

17.38b

collection. Many of the artists were acquaintances and neighbours of Hunter in Leicester Square or were part of Hunter's social set, which included scientists and explorers such as Sir Joseph Banks and Daniel Solander.

17.38

Hunter commissioned Rymsdyk to produce drawings for his publications. Rymsdyk is best known for illustrating William Hunter's *The Anatomy of the Human Gravid Uterus*, when John Hunter prepared the specimens, but John later commissioned Rymsdyk for his own work, including his first book *The Natural History of Teeth* (Fig 17.38a). As well as the delicate red chalk drawings, the collection includes a painting of a group of animals attributed to Rymsdyk by William Clift (Fig 17.38b).

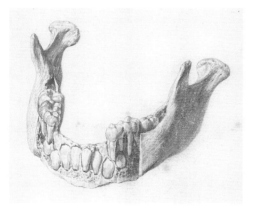

17.38a

17.39

John Hunter's drawing books have been conserved and stored in solander boxes so that they can be easily examined. They are a treasure chest for students of natural history and art as well as Hunter scholars. All kinds of fauna and flora were recorded at Hunter's behest; only a few of the drawings are signed by the artists, one of whom is Sawrey Gilpin (1733–1807), who specialised in animal (especially horse) paintings. Hunter was interested in breeding experiments and commissioned Gilpin to draw Mr Wright's Freemartin.

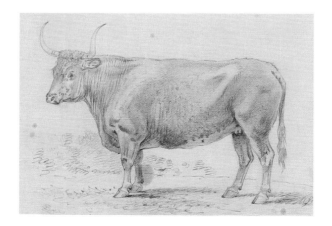

Specimen and Animal Portraits

In the 18th and 19th centuries anatomists and scientists pursued their studies through comparative anatomy and pathology. Scientific observations, experiments and treatments were recorded through art as in the Tonks drawings of facial injuries (see also Fig 15.18). Hunter's art collection includes important examples, but other items have come into the collection from this background. Joseph Lister was an accomplished draughtsman; the College's collection includes anatomical drawings (see also Fig 17.15) and sketches he made on country walks. Art is still used as one way of learning anatomy and as a means of recording cases.

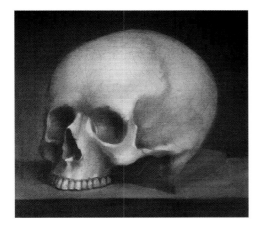

17.40

William Cheselden, a connoisseur of art and classical culture as well as a successful surgeon, painted a series of views of skulls. These paintings correspond to illustrations in Cheselden's major publication *Osteographia* in 1733.

17.41

William Clift and Sir Everard Home were extremely interested in the breeding experiments being carried out at the stable of The Earl of Morton, Vice-President of the Royal Society, during the 1820s and commissioned a series of six paintings from the Swiss animal painter Jacques Laurent Agasse (1767–1849). Eight further paintings of unusual or new species were added, possibly painted from examples brought over to England and kept in private menageries.

17.42

Sir Richard Owen, a surgeon, researcher and Conservator of the Hunterian Museum, recorded his dissections to show form and structure. This is a drawing of an apteryx.

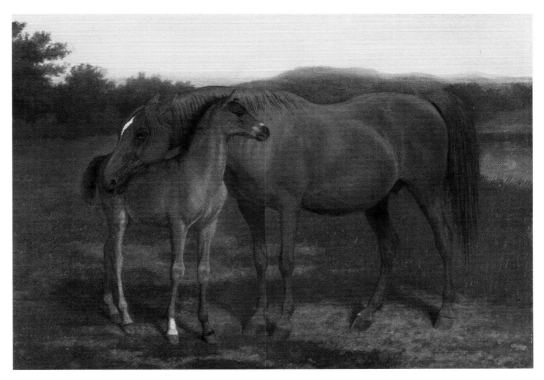

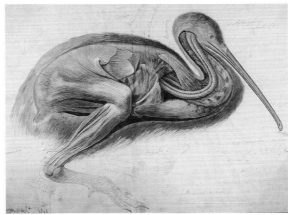

John Hunter

This statue is based on the Reynold's portrait (Fig 2.7). It was funded by public subscription and displayed in the Hunterian Museum. It was protected from damage during the Second World War and was moved to the Inner Hall in 1954.

By Henry Weeks, 1864

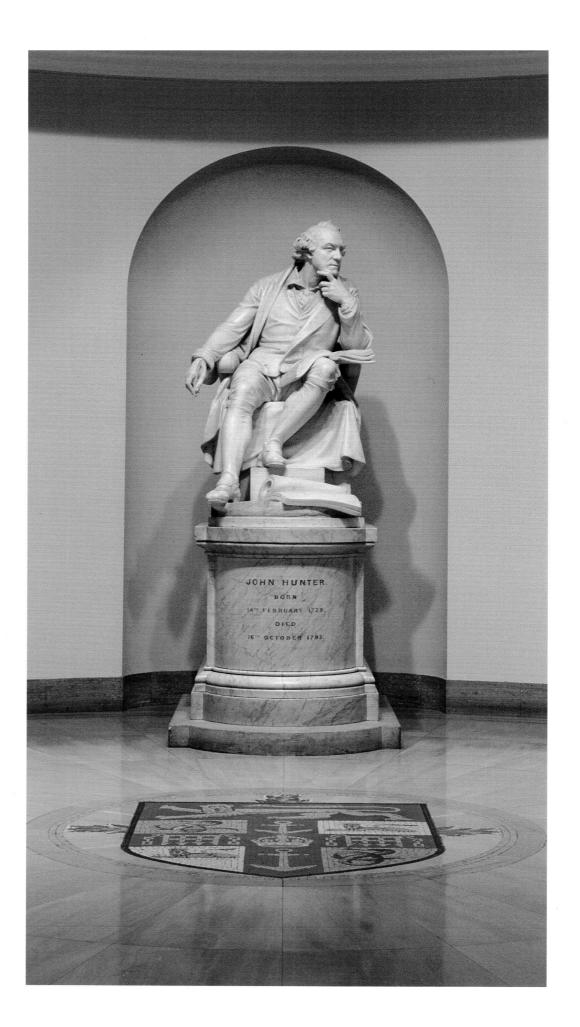

Masters

1799–1800	Charles Hawkins
1800	William Long
1801	George Chandler
1802	Thomas Keate
1803	Sir Charles Blicke
1804	David Dundas
1805	Thompson Forster
1806	Charles Hawkins
1807	Sir James Earle
1808	George Chandler
1809	Thomas Keate
1810	Sir Charles Blicke
1811	David Dundas
1812	Thompson Forster
1813	Sir Everard Home
1814	Sir William Blizard
1815	Henry Cline
1816	William Norris
1817	Sir James Earle/George Chandler
1818	Thomas Keate
1819	Sir David Dundas
1820	Thompson Forster
1821	Sir Everard Home

Presidents

1822	Sir Everard Home/Sir William Blizard
1823	Henry Cline
1824	William Norris
1825	William Lynn
1826	John Abernethy
1827	Sir Astley Paston Cooper
1828	Sir Anthony Carlisle
1829	Honoratus Leigh Thomas
1830	Richard Clement Headington
1831	Robert Keate
1832	John Painter Vincent
1833	George James Guthrie
1834	Anthony White
1835	John Goldwyer Andrews
1836	Sir Astley Paston Cooper
1837	Sir Anthony Carlisle
1838	Honoratus Leigh Thomas
1839	Robert Keate
1840	John Painter Vincent
1841	George James Guthrie
1842	Anthony White
1843	John Goldwyer Andrews
1844	Sir Benjamin Collins Brodie
1845	Samuel Cooper
1846	William Lawrence
1847	Benjamin Travers
1848	Edward Stanley
1849	Joseph Henry Green
1850	James Moncrieff Arnott
1851	John Flint South
1852	Caesar Henry Hawkins
1853	James Luke
1854	George James Guthrie
1855	William Lawrence
1856	Benjamin Travers
1857	Edward Stanley
1858	Joseph Henry Green
1859	James Moncrieff Arnott
1860	John Flint South
1861	Caesar Henry Hawkins
1862	James Luke
1863	Frederic Carpenter Skey
1864	Joseph Hodgson
1865	Thomas Wormald
1866	Richard Partridge
1867	John Hilton
1868	Richard Quain
1869	Edward Cock
1870	Sir William Fergusson
1871	George Busk
1872	Henry Hancock
1873	Thomas Blizard Curling
1874	Frederick Le Gros Clark
1875	Sir James Paget
1876	Prescott Gardner Hewett
1877	John Birkett
1878	John Simon
1879	Luther Holden
1880	John Eric Erichsen

1881	Sir William James Erasmus Wilson
1882	Sir Thomas Spencer Wells
1883	John Marshall
1884	John Cooper Forster
1885–88	Sir William Scovell Savory
1889	Sir Jonathan Hutchinson
1890–92	Thomas Bryant
1893–94	John Whitaker Hulke
1895	Christopher Heath
1896–1900	Sir William MacCormac
1901–02	Sir Henry Greenway Howse
1903–05	Sir John Tweedy
1906–08	Sir Henry Morris
1909–11	Sir Henry Trentham Butlin
1911–13	Sir Rickman John Godlee
1914–16	Sir William Watson Cheyne
1917–19	Sir George Henry Makins
1920–22	Sir Anthony Alfred Bowlby
1923–25	Sir John Bland-Sutton
1926–31	Lord Moynihan
1932–34	Sir Holburt Jacob Waring
1935–37	Sir Cuthbert Sidney Wallace
1938–40	Sir Hugh Lett
1941–48	Lord Webb-Johnson
1949–53	Sir Cecil Pembrey Grey Wakeley
1954–56	Sir Harry Platt
1957–59	Sir James Paterson Ross
1960–62	Lord Porritt
1963–65	Lord Brock
1966–69	Sir Hedley John Barnard Atkins
1969–71	Sir Thomas Holmes Sellors
1972	Sir Edward Grainger Muir
1973–76	Lord Smith
1977–79	Sir Reginald Sydney Murley
1980–81	Sir Alan Parks
1982–85	Sir Geoffrey Slaney
1986–88	Sir Ian Todd
1989–91	Sir Terence English
1992–94	Sir Norman Browse
1995–97	Sir Rodney Sweetnam
1998–	Barry Jackson

Vice-Presidents

1822	Sir William Blizard	1851	Caesar Henry Hawkins	1880	Sir William James Erasmus Wilson
	Henry Cline		James Luke		Sir Thomas Spencer Wells
	William Norris	1852	James Luke	1881	Sir Thomas Spencer Wells
1823-24	Sir Ludford Harvey		Robert Keate		John Marshall
	William Lynn	1853	George James Guthrie	1882	John Marshall
1825	John Abernethy		William Lawrence		John Cooper Forster
	Sir Astley Paston Cooper	1854	William Lawrence	1883	John Cooper Forster
1826	Sir Anthony Carlisle		Benjamin Travers		Sir William Scovell Savory
	Sir Astley Paston Cooper	1855	Benjamin Travers	1884	Sir William Scovell Savory
1827	Sir Anthony Carlisle		Edward Stanley		Timothy Holmes
	Honoratus Leigh Thomas	1856	Edward Stanley	1885	John Wood
1828	Sir Patrick Macgregor		Joseph Henry Green		Henry Power
	Honoratus Leigh Thomas	1857	Joseph Henry Green	1886	Sir Jonathan Hutchinson
	Richard Headington		James Moncrieff Arnott		Lord Lister
1829	Robert Keate	1858	James Moncrieff Arnott	1887	Thomas Bryant
	Richard Headington		John Flint South		Thomas Smith
1830	John Painter Vincent	1859	John Flint South	1888	John Whitaker Hulke
	Robert Keate		Caesar Henry Hawkins		Christopher Heath
1831	George James Guthrie	1860	Caesar Henry Hawkins	1889	Thomas Bryant
	John Painter Vincent		James Luke		John Croft
1832	Anthony White	1861	James Luke	1890	Thomas Smith
	George James Guthrie		Frederic Carpenter Skey		Sir William MacCormac
1833	John Goldwyer Andrews	1862	Frederic Carpenter Skey	1891	John Whitaker Hulke
	Anthony White		Joseph Hodgson		Berkeley Hill
1834	Sir William Blizard	1863	Joseph Hodgson		Arthur Edward Durham
	John Goldwyer Andrews		Thomas Wormald	1892	Christopher Heath
	Sir Astley Paston Cooper	1864	Thomas Wormald		Arthur Edward Durham
1835	Sir Anthony Carlisle		Francis Kiernan	1893	Sir William MacCormac
	Sir Astley Paston Cooper	1865	Richard Partridge		Nottidge Charles Macnamara
1836	Sir Anthony Carlisle		John Hilton	1894	Reginald Hardson
	W Thomas	1866	John Hilton		Alfred Willett
1837	W Thomas		Richard Quain	1895	Reginald Harrison
	Robert Keate	1867	Richard Quain		Thomas Pickering Pick
1838	W Thomas		Edward Cock	1896	Nottidge Charles Macnamara
	Robert Keate	1868	Edward Cock		John Langton
1839	John Painter Vincent		Samuel Solly	1897	Alfred Willett
	George James Guthrie	1869	Samuel Solly		Sir Henry Greenway Howse
1840	George James Guthrie		Sir William Fergusson	1898	Thomas Pickering Pick
	Anthony White	1870	George Busk		Frederick Howard Marsh
1841	Anthony White		Henry Hancock	1899	Sir Henry Greenway Howse
	John Goldwyer Andrews	1871	Henry Hancock		Sir John Tweedy
1842	John Goldwyer Andrews		Thomas Blizard Curling	1900	John Langton
	Sir Benjamin Brodie	1872	Thomas Blizard Curling		Sir Henry Morris
1843	Sir Benjamin Brodie		Frederick Le Gros Clark	1901	Thomas Richard Jessop
	Samuel Cooper	1873	Frederick Le Gros Clark		Frederick Howard Marsh
1844	Samuel Cooper		Sir James Paget	1902	Sir John Tweedy
	William Lawrence	1874	Sir James Paget		Sir Arthur William Mayo Robson
1845	Benjamin Travers		Prescott Gardner Hewett	1903	Sir Henry Morris
	William Lawrence	1875	Prescott Gardner Hewett		Sir Alfred Cooper
1846	Benjamin Travers		John Birkett	1904	Arthur William Mayo Robson
	Edward Stanley	1876	John Birkett		Sir Henry Trentham Butlin
1847	Edward Stanley		John Simon	1905	Sir Henry Trentham Butlin
	Joseph Henry Green	1877	John Simon		Edmund Owen
1848	James Moncrieff Arnott		Luther Holden	1906	Edmund Owen
	Joseph Henry Green	1878	Luther Holden		Sir Rickman John Godlee
1849	James Moncrieff Arnott		John Erichsen	1907	Sir Rickman John Godlee
	John Flint South	1879	John Erichsen		Sir William Watson Cheyne
1850	John Flint South		Sir William James Erasmus Wilson	1908	Sir William Watson Cheyne
	Caesar Henry Hawkins				Alfred Leslie Pearce Gould

1909	Alfred Leslie Pearce Gould	1938	George Grey Turner	1968	Harold Clifford Edwards
	Richard Clement Lucas		Sir Robert Ernest Kelly		Sir Thomas Holmes Sellors
1910	Richard Clement Lucas	1939	Sir Robert Ernest Kelly	1969	Sir Frank Wild Holdsworth
	Charles William Mansell Moullin		Sir James Walton		Robert Victor Cooke
1911	Charles William Mansell Moullin	1940	Sir James Walton	1970	Sir Henry Osmond-Clarke
	Clinton Thomas Dent		Lord Webb-Johnson	1971	Norman Leslie Capener
1912	Clinton Thomas Dent	1941-42	Sir Gordon Gordon-Taylor		Sir Edward Grainger Muir
	Sir George Henry Makins		Leonard Ralph Braithwaite	1972	Norman Leslie Capener
	Edmund Owen	1943	Sir Henry Sessions Souttar		Norman Birkett
1913	Sir George Henry Makins		Sir William Girling Ball	1973	Norman Birkett
	Sir Frederic Samuel Eve	1944	Sir William Girling Ball		Alphonsus Liguori d'Abreu
1914	Sir Frederic Samuel Eve		Sir Charles Max Page	1974-75	Richard Harrington Franklin
	Sir Anthony Alfred Bowlby	1945	Sir Charles Max Page		Richard Sampson Handley
1915	Sir Frederic Samuel Eve		Sir William Heneage Ogilvie	1976	Selwyn Francis Taylor
	William Harrison Cripps	1946	Sir William Heneage Ogilvie		Walpole Sinclair Lewin
1916	William Harrison Cripps		Sir Cecil Pembrey Grey Wakeley	1977	Selwyn Francis Taylor
	Sir Charters James Symonds	1947	Sir Cecil Pembrey Grey Wakeley		Sir James Gordon Robson
1917	Sir Charters James Symonds		Lionel Edward Close Norbury	1978	Walpole Sinclair Lewin
	William Frederic Haslam	1948	Lionel Edward Close Norbury		Sir James Gordon Robson
1918	William Frederic Haslam		Sir Vincent Zachary Cope	1979	Howard Granville Hanley
	Sir John Bland-Sutton	1949	Sir Harry Platt		Sir Alan Parks
1919	Sir Anthony Alfred Bowlby		Sir Ernest Frederick Finch	1980	Howard Granville Hanley
	Sir John Bland-Sutton	1950	Sir Ernest Frederick Finch		Peter Gilroy Bevan
1920	Sir Charles Alfred Ballance		Philip Henry Mitchiner	1981	Peter Gilroy Bevan
	Sir John Bland-Sutton	1951	Philip Henry Mitchiner		Harry Hubert Grayson Eastcott
1921	Sir Charles Alfred Balance		Sir James Paterson Ross	1982	Harry Hubert Grayson Eastcott
	Sir D'Arcy Power	1952	Sir James Paterson Ross		Geoffrey John Hadfield
1922	Sir D'Arcy Power		Sir Reginald Watson-Jones	1983	Anthony John Harding Rains
	Lord Moynihan	1953	Sir Reginald Watson-Jones		Sir David Innes Williams
1923	Lord Moynihan		Lambert Charles Rogers	1984	Sir David Innes Williams
	Sir Holburt Jacob Waring	1954	Lambert Charles Rogers		Alan Graham Apley
1924	Sir Holburt Jacob Waring		Julian Taylor	1985	Harold Ellis
	Walter George Spencer	1955	Julian Taylor		Sir Donald Campbell
1925	Walter George Spencer		Robert Paul Scott Mason	1986	Sir Donald Campbell
	James Sherren	1956	Arthur Lawrence Abel		Peter Herent Lord
1926	Sir Cuthbert Sidney Wallace		Lord Brock	1987	Peter Herent Lord
	Francis James Steward	1957	Lord Brock		Sir Roy Yorke Calne
1927	Sir Cuthbert Sidney Wallace		Sir Archibald McIndoe	1988	Sir Roy Yorke Calne
	Francis James Steward	1958	Sir Archibald McIndoe		Phyllis Ann George
1928	Ernest William Hey Groves		Arthur Dickson Wright	1989	Phyllis Ann George
	Vincent Warren Low	1959	Arthur Dickson Wright		David Evans
1929	Charles Herbert Fagge		Sir Stanford Cade	1990	David Evans
	Vincent Warren Low	1960	Sir Stanford Cade		Jeffrey Adrian Priestley Marston
1930	Charles Herbert Fagge		Digby Chamberlain	1991	Jeffrey Adrian Priestley Marston
	Robert Pugh Rowlands	1961	Digby Chamberlain		John Rayne
1931	Robert Pugh Rowlands		Sir Eric William Riches	1992-93	Sir Rodney Sweetnam
	William Sampson Handley	1962	Sir Eric William Riches		John Peter Blandy
1932	William Sampson Handley		Sir Clement Price Thomas	1994	John Alexander-Williams
	Sir Percy Sargent	1963	Sir Clement Price Thomas		Alan William Frederick Lettin
1933	George Ernest Gask		Sir Clifford Naunton Morgan	1995	Alan William Frederick Lettin
	Wilfred Trotter	1964	Sir Clifford Naunton Morgan		Jack Donald Hardcastle
1934	Wilfred Trotter		Sir Hedley John Barnard Atkins	1996	Jack Donald Hardcastle
	Arthur Henry Burgess	1965	Sir Hedley John Barnard Atkins		Richard John Heald
1935	Arthur Henry Burgess		Charles Alexander Wells	1997	Richard John Heald
	Sir Charles Gordon-Watson	1966	Charles Alexander Wells		John Llewellyn Williams
1936	Sir Charles Gordon-Watson		Robert Milnes Walker	1998	John Llewellyn Williams
	Victor Bonney	1967	Robert Milnes Walker		Averil Olive Mansfield
1937	Victor Bonney		Harold Clifford Edwards	1999	Averil Olive Mansfield
	George Grey Turner				Charles Samuel Bernard Galasko

Court of Assistants

1800–13	Charles Hawkins
1800–18	William Long
1800–22	George Chandler
1800–01	Joseph Warner
1800–01	Samuel Howard
1800–01	William Cooper
1800–05	Jonathan Wathen
1800–10	William Lucas
1800–17	Sir James Earle
1800–15	Sir Charles Blicke
1800–27	Thompson Forster
1800–15	John Birch
1800–21	Thomas Keate
1800–28	John Heaviside
1800–08	John Howard
1800–35	Sir William Blizard
1800–27	Henry Cline
1800–26	Sir David Dundas
1800–16	John Samuel Charlton
1800–10	Edward Ford
1800–27	William Norris
1801–15	James Ware
1801–27	Sir Everard Home
1805–32	John Adair Hawkins
1808–27	Francis Knight
1810–27	Sir Ludford Harvey
1810–35	William Lynn
1810–30	John Abernethy
1813–30	William Lucas
1815–41	Sir Astley Paston Cooper
1815–40	Sir Anthony Carlisle
1816–17	Thomas Blizard
1816–24	Thomas Chevalier
1817–21	James Wilson
1817–24	John Gunning
1818–45	Honoratus Leigh Thomas
1821–31	Richard Clement Headington
1822–57	Robert Keate

Council Members

1822–51	John Painter Vincent
1824–56	George James Guthrie
1824–29	William Wadd
1826–28	Sir Patrick Macgregor
1827–30	Henry Jeffreys
1827–46	Anthony White
1827–49	John Goldwyer Andrews
1827–48	Samuel Cooper
1827–54	Thomas Copeland
1828–41	John Howship
1828–48	James Briggs
1828–67	Sir William Lawrence
1829–62	Sir Benjamin Collins Brodie
1830–58	Benjamin Travers
1830–38	Henry Earle
1830–38	Sir Charles Bell
1831–70	Joseph Swan
1832–62	Edward Stanley
1835–63	Joseph Henry Green
1835–48	Thomas Callaway
1836–45	George Gisborne Babington
1838–43	Frederick Tyrrell
1840–47	Robert Liston
1841–65	James Moncrieff Arnott
1841–73	John Flint South
1843–47	John Morgan
1844–49	Richard Wellbank
1844–46	John Scott
1844–51	Edward Cutler
1845–49	Charles Aston Key
1846–63	Caesar Henry Hawkins
1846–50	Richard Dugard Grainger
1846–66	James Luke
1848–67	Frederic Carpenter Skey
1848–52	Richard Anthony Stafford
1848–53	Bransby Blake Cooper
1849–68	Joseph Hodgson
1849–67	Thomas Wormald
1849–55	George Pilcher
1849–61	John Bishop
1850–69	Gilbert Wakefield Mackmurdo
1850–67	Francis Kiernan
1851–63	William Coulson
1851–52	John Dalrymple
1852–64	George Gulliver
1852–68	Richard Partridge
1854–78	John Hilton
1854–73	Richard Quain
1856–71	Edward Cock
1856–72	Samuel Solly
1857–63	Thomas Tatum
1858–65	Alexander Shaw
1861–77	Sir William Fergusson
1862–70	Thomas Paget
1862–65	John Adams
1863–71	Samuel Armstrong Lane
1863–80	George Busk
1863–80	Henry Hancock
1864–80	Thomas Blizard Curling

1864–79	Frederick Le Gros Clark
1865–73	Thomas Turner
1865–89	Sir James Paget
1866–73	Charles Hawkins
1867–83	Sir Prescott Gardner Hewett
1867–75	Henry Spencer Smith
1867–83	John Birkett
1868–80	Sir John Simon
1868–84	Sir George Murray Humphry
1868–84	Luther Holden
1869–77	John Gay
1869–85	Sir John Eric Erichsen
1870–84	Sir Wm. Jas. Erasmus Wilson
1870–78	Henry Lee
1871–95	Sir Thomas Spencer Wells
1871–79	George Critchett
1872–78	Barnard Wight Holt
1873–81	Haynes Walton
1873–90	John Marshall
1873–76	George Southam
1874–82	Alfred Baker
1875–86	John Cooper Forster
1876–81	Claudius Galen Wheelhouse
1877–93	Sir William Scovell Savory
1877–85	Timothy Holmes
1878–84	John Gay
1878–94	Edward Lund
1879–87	John Wood
1879–90	Henry Power
1879–95	Sir Jonathan Hutchinson
1880–95	William Cadge
1880–85	Lord Lister
1880–1904	Thomas Bryant
1880–1900	Sir Thomas Smith
1881–95	John Whitaker Hulke
1881–97	Christopher Heath
1882–90	John Croft
1883–91	Sydney Jones
1883–1901	Sir William MacCormac
1884–86	William Allingham
1884–92	George Lawson
1884–92	Matthew Berkeley Hill
1884–95	Arthur Edward Durham
1885–1901	Nottidge Charles Macnamara
1885–97	Oliver Pemberton
1886–91	Septimus William Sibley
1886–1902	Reginald Harrison
1887–1903	Alfred Willett
1888–1903	Thomas Pickering Pick
1889–1905	Sir Henry Greenway Howse
1890–1906	John Langton
1890–93	Marcus Beck
1890–98	Sir William Mitchell Banks
1891–97	Walter Rivington
1891–1903	Thomas Richard Jessop
1892–1908	Frederick Howard Marsh
1892–1907	Sir John Tweedy
1893–1914	Sir Henry Morris
1893–1909	Sir Arthur William Mayo Robson

1894–1902	James Hardie	1923–31	John Herbert Fisher	1953–62	Ian Aird
1895–99	John Ward Cousins	1923–45	William Sampson Handley	1955–63	Ronald Henry Ottywell Betham Robinson
1895–1905	Sir Alfred Cooper	1923–33	Sir Percy Sargent	1955–71	Harold Clifford Edwards
1895–1912	Sir Henry Trentham Butlin	1923–39	George Ernest Gask	1957–65	Francis Roland Stammers
1895–1903	Sir Frederick Treves	1924–32	William McAdam Eccles	1957–73	Sir Thomas Holmes Sellors
1896–1900	John Neville Colley Davies-Colley	1924–39	Wilfred Trotter	1958–66	John Cridlan Barrett
1897–1913	Edmund Owen	1924–32	Sir Charles Gordon-Watson	1958–66	Sir Frank Wild Holdsworth
1897–1915	Sir Rickman John Godlee	1925–48	Arthur Henry Burgess	1959–75	Robert Victor Cooke
1897–1918	Sir William Watson Cheyne	1926–33	Vincent Warren Low	1959–75	Sir Henry Osmond-Clarke
1898–1914	Francis Richardson Cross	1926–46	Victor Bonney	1960–68	Leslie Norman Pyrah
1899–1907	Herbert William Page	1926–50	George Grey Turner	1961–69	Norman Leslie Capener
1900–08	John Ward Cousins	1927–43	Sir Hugh Lett	1961–69	Sir Edward Grainger Muir
1900–16	Sir Alfred P. Gould	1928–35	Leonard Parker Gamgee	1963–71	Norman Rupert Barrett
1901–14	Richard Clement Lucas	1928–36	Robert George Hogarth	1963–71	Norman Cecil Tanner
1902–10	John Hammond Morgan	1928–44	Sir Robert Ernest Kelly	1963–71	Alphonsus Liguori d'Abreu
1902–10	Henry Hugh Clutton	1929–39	Graham Scales Simpson	1963–71	Alexander William Badenoch
1902–15	Charles William Mansell Moullin	1931–47	Sir Albert James Walton	1964–72	Harold Jackson Burrows
1903–12	Clinton Thomas Dent	1932–50	Lord Webb-Johnson	1965–77	Richard Harrington Franklin
1903–21	Sir George Henry Makins	1932–48	Sir Gordon Gordon-Taylor	1965–70	Alan Henderson Hunt
1904–16	Sir Frederic Samuel Eve	1933–40	Sir Charles Gordon-Watson	1965–78	Lord Smith
1904–27	Sir Anthony Alfred Bowlby	1933–40	Reginald Cheyne Elmslie	1966–78	Richard Sampson Handley
1904–12	Sir Harry Gilbert Barling	1933–42	Leonard Ralph Braithwaite	1966–78	Selwyn Francis Taylor
1905–13	Cuthbert Hilton Golding-Bird	1933–49	Sir Henry Sessions Souttar	1966–70	Eric Leslie Farquharson
1905–08	William Harrison Cripps	1934–45	Sir William Girling Ball	1967–79	George Qvist
1906–10	George Arthur Wright	1935–43	Seymour Gilbert Barling	1968–76	Ronald William Raven
1907–13	William Bruce Clarke	1936–52	Sir Charles Max Page	1968–80	John Cedric Goligher
1907–23	Sir Charters James Symonds	1936–52	Sir William Heneage Ogilvie	1969–81	David Trevor
1908–24	William Frederic Haslam	1937–55	Sir Cecil Pembrey Grey Wakeley	1969–81	Howard Granville Hanley
1908–14	Charles Barlett Lockwood	1938–53	Lionel Edward Close Norbury	1970–80	Walpole Sinclair Lewin
1908–16	Sir William Arbuthnot Lane	1939–47	Robert Joseph Willan	1970–82	Sir Reginald Sydney Murley
1909–20	William Harrison Cripps	1939–45	Cecil Augustus Joll	1971–83	Harry Hubert Grayson Eastcott
1910–18	Bilton Pollard	1940–49	Sir Vincent Zachary Cope	1971–83	Geoffrey John Hadfield
1910–26	Sir Charles Alfred Balance	1940–58	Sir Harry Platt	1971–83	Sir Alan Guyatt Parks
1910–27	Sir John Bland-Sutton	1941–57	Sir Ernest Frederick Finch	1971–83	Peter Gilroy Bevan
1912–28	Sir D'Arcy Power	1942–50	Sir Hugh William Bell Cairns	1971–83	Sir John Cecil Nicholson Wakeley
1912–33	Lord Moynihan	1943–52	Philip Henry Mitchiner	1972–84	Anthony John Harding Rains
1913–21	James Ernest Lane	1943–46	Arthur Tudor Edwards	1973–85	Alan Graham Apley
1913–18	Louis Albert Dunn	1943–61	Sir James Paterson Ross	1973–85	Michael Charles Tempest Reilly
1913–14	Jonathan Hutchinson	1943–59	Sir Reginald Watson-Jones	1974–86	Sir David Innes Williams
1913–37	Sir Holburt Jacob Waring	1943–59	Lambert Charles Rogers	1974–86	Harold Ellis
1914–16	James Stanley Newton Boyd	1944–52	Sir Geoffrey Langton Keynes	1974–86	Ivan David Alexander Johnston
1914–23	Sir William Thorburn	1945–53	Robert John McNeill Love	1975–87	Sir Ian Pelham Todd
1914–22	William McAdam Eccles	1946–62	Julian Taylor	1975–87	Sir Geoffrey Slaney
1914–22	Sir Charles Ryall	1946–56	Robert Paul Scott Mason	1976–84	George Charles Lloyd-Roberts
1915–26	Walter George Spencer	1947–63	Arthur Lawrence Abel	1977–82	John Bernard Kinmonth
1915–23	Frédéric François Burghard	1947–55	James Bagot Oldham	1977–80	Kenneth Peters Liddelow
1915–23	Sir Herbert Furnivall Waterhouse	1948–67	Lord Brock	1977–81	Sir James Gordon Robson
1916–24	Thomas Horrocks Openshaw	1948–60	Sir Archibald Hector McIndoe	1977–79	John Edmund Riding
1916–24	Raymond Johnson	1949–65	Arthur Dickson Wright	1977–82	John Francis Nunn
1916–25	Vincent Warren Low	1949–65	Sir Stanford Cade	1977–78	Geoffrey Leslie Howe
1917–26	James Sherren	1949–62	Digby Chamberlain	1977–79	Ivor Robert Horton Kramer
1918–33	Sir John Lynn-Thomas	1950–58	Angus Hedley Whyte	1977–79	Paul Anthony Bramley
1918–42	Ernest William Hey Groves	1950–66	Sir Eric William Riches	1978–86	James Stanley Hilary Wade
1919–43	Sir Cuthbert Sidney Wallace	1950–66	Lord Porritt	1978–86	Peter Herent Lord
1920–36	Francis James Steward	1952–64	Sir Clement Price Thomas	1978–86	Sir Roy Yorke Calne
1921–27	William Thelwall Thomas	1952–68	Sir Clifford Naunton Morgan	1979–81	Douglas Donald Currie Howat
1921–38	Charles Herbert Fagge	1952–68	Sir Hedley John Barnard Atkins	1979–87	Phyllis Ann George
1922–33	Robert Pugh Rowlands	1953–69	Charles Alexander Wells	1980–88	William John Wells Sharrard
1923–29	Sir James Berry	1953–69	Robert Milnes Walker	1980–82	David Downton

1980–88	Richard Trevor Turner–Warwick	1995–	Hugh Phillips
1980–84	Roy Duckworth	1995–	Peter Leopard
1981–89	Terence Leslie Kennedy	1996–	Thomas Treasure
1981–84	Michael Douglas Allen Vickers	1996–	Anne Moore
1981–84	Sir Donald Campbell	1996–97	John K Williams
1981–89	Sir Terence Alexander Hawthorne English	1997–98	Bernard Smith
1982–83	Ian Hanson Heslop	1998–	Bernard Ribeiro
1982–84	Aileen Kirkpatrick Adams	1998–	Michael Bishop
1982–94	John Peter Blandy	1998–	David Barnard
1983–91	David Lawrence Evans	1999–	Ronald Christopher Gordon Russell
1983–91	Anthony Hugh Cyril Ratliff	1999–	Linda de Cossart
1983–92	Robert Owen		
1983–84	Gordon Robert Seward		
1983–95	John Alexander–Williams		
1983–91	Raymond Maurice Kirk		
1983–92	John Rayne		
1983–95	Sir Miles Horsfall Irving		
1984–96	Alan William Frederick Lettin		
1984–92	Philip Metcalfe Yeoman		
1984–86	Derek Henderson		
1984–88	Richard Stuart Atkinson		
1985–88	Aileen Kirkpatrick Adams		
1985–98	Sir David Rodney Sweetnam		
1985–95	Jeffrey Adrian Priestley Marston		
1986–90	Gordon Robert Seward		
1986–98	Hugh Brendan Devlin		
1986–88	Peter Wentworth Thompson		
1986–95	Sir Norman Leslie Browse		
1986–94	Sir Keith James Ross		
1986–94	Lord McColl		
1987–92	Derek Seel		
1987–99	Jack Donald Hardcastle		
1988–91	Michael Rosen		
1988–90	John Stanley Mornington Zorab		
1988–94	Alastair Andrew Spence		
1989–	Richard John Heald		
1989–96	Brian McKibbin		
1990–	Thomas Duckworth		
1990–	Averil Olive Mansfield		
1990–95	Kenneth Richard Ray		
1991–	Sir Peter John Morris		
1991–	Charles Samuel Bernard Galasko		
1991–99	Brian David Gwynne Morgan		
1991–	Barry Trevor Jackson		
1991–92	David John Hatch		
1992–	George Bentley		
1992–96	Joseph Dermot Strahan		
1992–	John Arthur Shenthall Carruth		
1992–	Leela Kapila		
1992–	Peter Robert Frank Bell		
1992–94	Peter Banks		
1993–	Peter Cameron May		
1994–	Valerie Joan Lund		
1994–	David James Dandy		
1994–	Richard David Rosin		
1994–	John Llewellyn Williams		
1995–	John Stuart Penton Lumley		
1995–	Michael Alan Edgar		
1995–	Charles David Collins		

Further Reading

Bailey H, Bishop WJ. *Notable Names in Medicine and Surgery*. London: HK Lewis; 1959.

Beck RT. *The Cutting Edge. Early History of the Surgeons of London*. London: Lund Humphries; 1974.

Bynum WF, Porter R (Eds). *Companion Encyclopaedia of the History of Medicine*. London: Routledge; 1993.

Cope, Z. *The Royal College of Surgeons of England, A History*. London: Blond; 1959.

Dobson J, Milnes Walker R. *Barbers and Barber-Surgeons of London*. Oxford: Blackwell Scientific Publications; 1979.

Haeger K. *The Illustrated History of Surgery*. London: Harold Starke; 1988.

LeFanu W. *A Catalogue of the Portraits and Other Paintings, Drawings and Sculptures in the Royal College of Surgeons of England*. London: Livingstone; 1960.

Negus VE. *Artistic Possessions at The Royal College of Surgeons of England*. London: Livingstone; 1967.

Rutkow IM. *Surgery; An Illustrated History*. Baltimore: Mosby-Year Book Inc.; 1993.

Sournia J-C. *The Illustrated History of Medicine*. London: Harold Starke; 1992.

Qvist G. *John Hunter 1728–1793*. London: Heinemann; 1981.

Wall C. *The History of the Surgeons' Company 1745–1800*. London: Hutchinson; 1937.

Webber, Wilfred. (1997) *The History of the Royal College of Surgeons of England 1959–1995*. Unpublished manuscript.

Acknowledgements

John Carruth, Chairman of the Bicentenary History Book Committee

Authors of Chapters

Aileen Adams, Helen Allgrove, John Blandy, Norman Browse, Jack Hardcastle, Thalia Knight, John Lumley, Stella Mason, Peter Morris, Malcolm Pendlebury, Karen Smith, John Ll Williams

Editorial Assistance

Peter Bell, Natalie Briggs, Bertram Cohen, Charles Collins, Martyn Coomer, Tina Craig, Alan Crockard, Roger Duffett, Craig Duncan, Mark Emberton, Jonathan Fountain, Jacqueline Fowler, Elizabeth Hoadley-Maidment, Barry Jackson, Andrea Kelly, John Kirkup, John McGhee, Peter Roberts, Sarah Robinson, Wilfrid Webber, Neil Weir

Production Team

Camilla Brandt, Jo Doyle, Carlos Sharpin, Caroline Williams, Jane Withey

Individuals Index

Subject Index